VEGANSTYLE

VEGANSTYLE

Your plant-based guide to
fashion + beauty + home + travel

SASCHA CAMILLI

TILLER PRESS

NEW YORK LONDON TORONTO SYDNEY NEW DELHI

CONTENTS

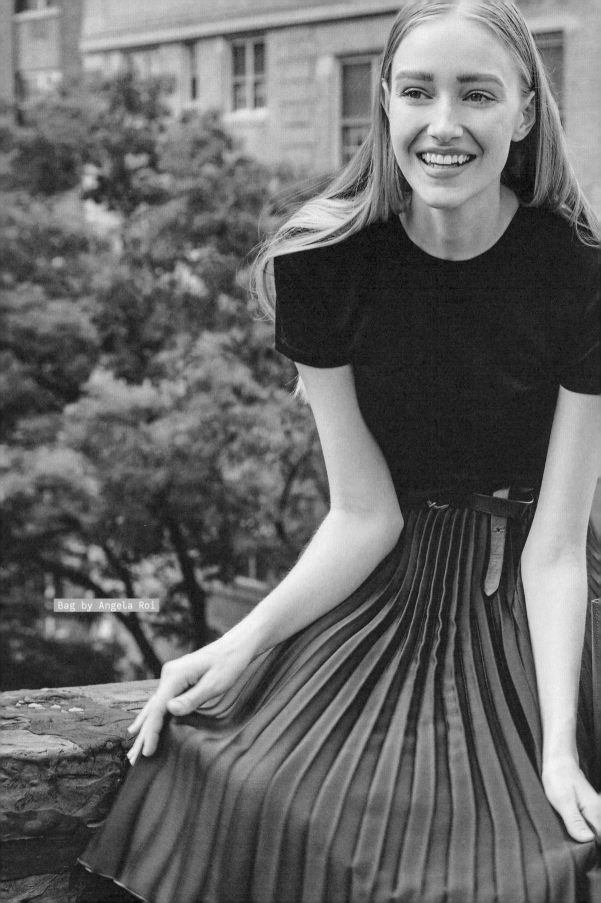

Bag by Angela Roi

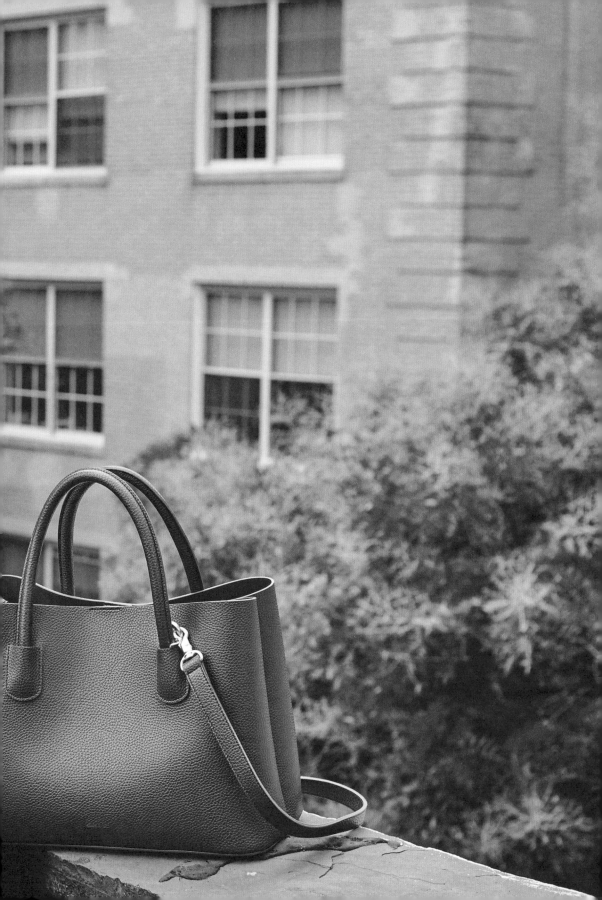

FOREWORD

Fashion can be a minefield for most women, let alone for a vegan individual in pursuit of a stylish and ethical lifestyle. Sascha's book is a joy, because it cuts through the fluff of regular fashion dialogue to guide even the most seasoned style lover to a well-thought-out and masterfully curated capsule wardrobe. It's well-researched, informative, and passionately communicates what it is to live a cruelty-free lifestyle, thoughtfully.

After twenty-five years as a magazine fashion director, I wish I'd had this little gem sooner. As a longtime vegetarian and new vegan, I find it invaluable, and it will be my constant companion on my continued journey to a kinder lifestyle.

SHELLY VELLA, AUGUST 2019

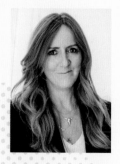

Shelly Vella is a former fashion director at Cosmopolitan UK *and winner of PETA UK's Innovation Award for her initiative to implement a no-fur and no-exotic-skins policy at the magazine. Shelly was also behind the 2005 Smart Girls Fake It pro-faux-fur campaign at* Cosmopolitan. *She is now a freelance fashion consultant.*

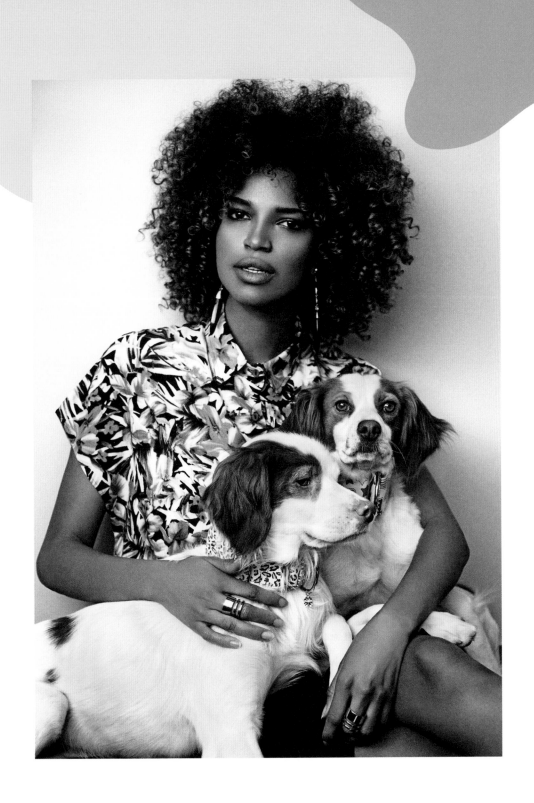

9

INTRODUCTION
What is vegan fashion, and why should you wear it?

I still remember the moment when I decided I wanted to work in fashion. The year was 2006, and a rather clueless twenty-two-year-old version of me was working on the shop floor of the Florence branch of an Italian lingerie chain called Yamamay. The post-Christmas sale attracted herds of customers every day, meaning we hardly had time to breathe, let alone think about what we wanted to do with the rest of our lives. We were selling garters and camisoles by the dozen, running up and down the stairs with heaps of bras in hand, smiling at customers, and expertly gift-wrapping lacy nighties.

One day, my very strict and demanding manager asked me to change the shop window. I viewed this as an invitation to fail, since she was the only person allowed to change it and did so about ten times a day, never satisfied. She was constantly contemplating the window, always finding something wrong with the fruits of her own labor. Undeterred, I played around with colors and shapes, pairing flirty undies with frilly bras. The window was my little masterpiece—but I knew it would soon be swapped for something that was more to the manager's taste.

The following morning, as we all gathered in front of the shop waiting for the manager to pull the key out of her Tod's bag and open up, I cast a quick glance at the window—and my creation was still there. It stayed untouched for several days.

That was the first time I took notice of how the juxtaposition of materials, textures, colors, and styles could create something that attracted people's attention. I was hooked. I wanted more. And so I continued exploring fashion, studying fashion, reading about fashion—immersing myself in it. I devoured fashion magazines and learned the names of fabrics, cuts, silhouettes, designers. Every

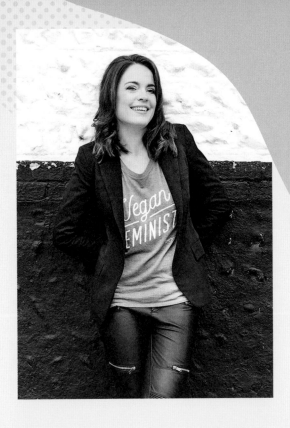

month, I waited eagerly for *Elle UK* to reach me in Italy, where I lived at the time, and read it from cover to cover before moving on to the next fashion bible.

A writer since I was a child, I became a freelance journalist and copywriter as soon as my days in the world of satin underwear were over. After working with five Swedish national women's magazines and a few Italian ones, I became a fashion editor for one of the world's biggest online retailers. Writing about clothes thrilled me, as what people buy is such an interesting mirror of society. What we wear reflects what's going on in the world—what we're doing, thinking, eating, listening to, and watching is reflected in our style choices. Fashion is in everything, as Coco Chanel used to say. And I was seeing it now more than ever. But, as I explored this new, all-consuming passion by working in the industry, I found that it was at odds with my lifestyle.

I went vegetarian at age eleven. People around me expected this to be a phase, but, nearly two decades later, at twenty-nine, I went vegan. I've always felt an attraction to a cruelty-free lifestyle, and after

INTRODUCTION

reading Jonathan Safran Foer's rather heartbreaking and very eye-opening *Eating Animals*, I found that I was constantly haunted by thoughts of all the animal cruelty that's inherent in society: from meat to leather to animal-tested household cleaning products. I couldn't find peace, as everything I touched seemed to be tainted with suffering. When I moved to London in 2012 and went vegan, it wasn't just about diet. My entire life was, slowly but surely, cleansed of cruel products, which gave my existence a whole new meaning—I'm not kidding. From the obvious health benefits of eating vegan—the stomachaches I'd been suffering from for years were long gone—to a higher emotional connection to everything I ate and wore, veganism resonated with me in a way that nothing ever had before. My wardrobe underwent a transformation: every new pair of shoes was leather-free (this was the glorious point in my life when I discovered Converse), and I explored the world of vegan cosmetics, which was much more exciting than I had expected it to be. After a few months, I had forgotten my old drugstore staples in favor of new, all-vegan brands. As my makeup cabinet shed its old skin, so did my mentality. Veganism had transformed me on a deep level—something that would also become clear in my work.

Working in fashion and leading a vegan lifestyle might seem like a contradiction, and, in fact, it was often questioned both by my industry peers and fellow vegans. How could I thrive in an industry that largely focuses on selling animal skins to people for large sums of money? The answer was, I couldn't. But there was a shift afoot, and many compassionate people were already working to bring consciousness to the mainstream fashion industry, known for its cruel and unethical practices. These people were willing to look behind the label, beyond the appearance, and start the discussion around ethical fashion. Accomplishing change is not easy, and baby steps are, in my opinion, the best—if not the only—way to go.

My own contribution to cruelty-free fashion is the digital magazine *Vilda* (which means "the wild one" in Swedish), which I created at the end of 2013 in collaboration with *Marie Claire* magazine's Inspire & Mentor scheme. Stylish, conscious, and informative, *Vilda* aims to showcase vegan brands in a beautiful way, conveying the infinite possibilities of cruelty-free style. I wanted to find new ways to present ethical brands—to give them the same creative and elevated exposure that mainstream brands get in magazines. And maybe attract a non-vegan reader or two, just to give them an insight into life on the cruelty-free side.

At the time of *Vilda*'s launch, there was already a bit of a discussion about ethical fashion, which I was excited about—until I found out that many new brands' definition of "ethical" included leather and wool: two cruel materials that are anything but ethical or sustainable. There was even talk of "ethical fur"—an oxymoron if ever I've heard one.

There is a lot of green-washing in the fashion industry—a common phenomenon where an industry or a company highlights a smaller practice or procedure that might be or seem eco-friendly in order to appear virtuous and divert attention from other practices that aren't as ethical. And it's not just among the fast-fashion brands. They are, of course, offenders—even if they offer vegan styles—but I often marvel at the sins that "luxury" fashion brands get away with. Sometimes, expensive brands are considered eco-friendlier because it's a common belief that their products will last longer, and, as a result, lessen the quantity of textiles thrown away, but that is not always the case. I have several cheap, non-designer finds that I've had for years, and they came from a thrift shop to begin with! Plus, luxury brands are often behind some of the most appalling animal cruelty in the industry, such as the slaughter of alligators, crocodiles, snakes, and ostriches for exotic-skin accessories with stratospheric price tags.

It's important to look behind the expensive exterior of luxury brands to see if their practices are truly more animal-friendly, or indeed human-friendly, than those of the much-blamed fast-fashion labels. Whether it's a luxury brand or a department store, animal cruelty must be taken into consideration. My stance is this: there is no humane way to kill an animal that wants to live. I don't care how much grass an animal has been fed, how many acres it has had to roam wild in—at the end of the day, you're still taking its life in the name of fashion. It's amazing how many people try to justify taking a life simply because, up until the killing point, the animal supposedly had a "good life." And with calfskin and lamb leather considered top choices for bags, that life can be heartbreakingly short.

There are myriad ways for us to improve the design and manufacturing processes of natural and man-made materials that could replace some of the animal products the fashion industry relies so heavily upon. And innovation is truly under way in this area—keep reading to find out more about exciting vegan and eco-fabrics.

I believe there is a bright, beautiful future for vegan fashion. A new crop of designers is innovating eco-friendly materials to create collections that rival traditional fashion—with a cruelty-free twist. *Vilda* was born out of the desire to bring animal-free fashion into the limelight and support these pioneers. Some of them prefer to keep their vegan lifestyle understated in their communication, while others proudly advertise their beliefs. Some create minimalist styles that slot seamlessly into the crowd at high-end fashion events, and others make high-quality sportswear to run or do yoga in. Some offer head-turning prints, while others go with sleek, clean-cut lines. Some create skyscraper heels, and others offer slouchy tote bags. But they have one thing in common: they want to use fashion to create a world where we all live in harmony (or get as close as we can, anyway). And I want to support them.

This book is intended to be an inspirational style guide for compassionate shoppers. It's a place where you can find the shopping inspiration that traditional magazines won't give you. This is a book that will explore vegan products, brands, and materials to give you insight and ideas. I hope you'll love reading it as much as I loved writing it.

Jascha Camilli

What do "vegan" and "cruelty-free" actually mean?

Throughout this book, I will use the terms "vegan" and "cruelty-free," and you might think that these terms are interchangeable. But, while they're closely linked, there is a slight distinction.

"Vegan" means that a product has no animal-derived ingredients. For food, which we won't cover much in this book (this is a kitchen-free zone!), this means no meat, fish, dairy, eggs, gelatin, or honey. Vegan fashion implies that a garment is free from fur, leather, wool, angora, exotic skins, mohair, silk, down, horn, or teeth (yep, some jewelry uses animal teeth). For beauty, there is a whole variety of ingredients that are animal-derived, and we cover them in chapter 4 (page 106), and a vegan home contains no leather sofas or wool/fur throws. All of these areas (and more) are covered in this book.

"Cruelty-free" is a term that's often used in reference to cosmetics and household products. What it means is that the finished product and its ingredients have not been tested on animals, by the company itself or any third parties.

A vegan product is often also cruelty-free, but there have been instances where cosmetic items have been marked as "vegan"—as they technically contained no animal-derived ingredients—but, as they had also been tested on animals, they could not qualify as cruelty-free.

A cruelty-free product that's not vegan is more common in cosmetics and household products. A lipstick that has carmine (actual crushed bugs; find out more in chapter 4) is, of course, not vegan, as bugs are animals. However, if the lipstick hasn't been tested on animals, it can be sold as cruelty-free.

FAS

A CRUELTY-FREE

HION
WARDROBE

Because animal skins are *so last* century.

Whenever I stumble across one of those magazine articles

along the lines of the "must-have pieces for every woman," my initial reaction is to partake in this ridiculous ticking off of items in my head: check, check, not check . . . before inevitably pausing to ponder what the world would look like if every woman wore similar clothing. If we all listen to this sort of advice, won't we all end up looking the same? I envision an army of ladies flicking their "carefree" ombré wavy hair around, in their "no makeup" makeup, before marching off down the street in their trench coats, carrying Birkin bags.

But there is a reason why jeans and trench coats keep ending up on those lists. The appeal of high-end basics with serious staying power is in their mix-and-match potential: a good pair of jeans, for example, looks effortlessly perfect with a slouchy T-shirt, as well as with a crisp blouse. They can be dressed down with sneakers or glammed up with stilettos. Once you've found The Pair, you'll live in them, and this holds true for the other "musts" as well. These pieces are reliable, versatile, and, if chosen well, will fit your body like a glove, meaning you'll get years out of them—years of creativity in styling them with accessories and more on-trend extras. Plus, as your style changes over time, you can adapt these pieces to any look, as they are evergreen classics.

Sweater by Armed
Angels, pants by
People Tree,
sneakers by Veja.
All from
Thrivestore.se.

What is a CAPSULE WARDROBE?

The term "capsule wardrobe" was coined by Susie Faux (love that vegan-friendly surname!), owner of London fashion boutique Wardrobe, in the 1970s. Her definition of a capsule wardrobe was a collection of garments that wouldn't go out of style and could be worn interchangeably and supplemented with seasonal pieces. Donna Karan subsequently released a capsule wardrobe collection of seven pieces in 1985.

More recently, the term has become a favorite of the sustainable fashion movement, as it minimizes the need to constantly acquire new garments and prolongs the lifespan of a so-called basic item that can be worn with anything in your wardrobe. The idea is to rely on fewer, more versatile items that can be used to build a variety of outfits. The important thing to keep in mind when building your capsule wardrobe is that it has to be useful and helpful to your lifestyle. So, before you start building it, take a look at your everyday life: What kind of clothes do you wear to work? How do you dress when relaxing and socializing? What seasonal items are needed? Build your wardrobe to fit your taste, personality, and lifestyle, and you'll never have an "I have nothing to wear!" morning again. (Well, almost never. Let's be realistic.)

Going back to those magazine articles, I notice that they focus heavily on animal-derived materials: "a cashmere sweater is worth the investment," "splurge on a handbag in long-lasting leather," and so on. It brings to mind all the things that are off-limits for me as a vegan. But that doesn't mean building a vegan capsule wardrobe is impossible. New, innovative materials make it possible to create clothing and accessories that will stand the test of time and last as long as their "finest" non-vegan counterparts. If we look at the capsule wardrobe from a sustainability angle, buying to last makes sense. This is primarily why I'm an avid supporter of the capsule wardrobe—it keeps our fashionista spirits from straining the Earth's resources.

(1) Virtually all winter coats are made with wool—and the few that aren't often contain synthetic materials treated with planet-harming chemicals.

(2) The same goes for knitwear. If it's not wool or angora (I feel my skin itching as I type the word "angora"), it's likely to be polyester.

The top five difficulties vegans face when shopping for basics

(3) Silk features heavily in the evening clutch department, especially if you're a fan of high-end designers.

(5) Even when you do find that elusive accessory in an animal-friendly material, you can't get your hopes up; more often than not there will be a leather trim, or it will have been pieced together with animal glue.

(4) Leather is pretty much synonymous with luxury when it comes to staple accessories: shoes, bags, wallets, and so on. But the tide is now turning toward good-quality, cruelty-free accessories.

FASHION

WHAT'S IN A LABEL?
a crash course in clothing-label reading for vegans

If you've already tried following a vegan diet, you will be familiar with label reading. That little piece of information that you might never have considered before cutting animal-derived ingredients from your life has now become all-important: after all, the label has the power to tell you whether you can use that product at all or not, so checking before you buy is crucial. Look out for the following words on your clothing labels and avoid them if you're aiming to shop vegan.

LEATHER

Most words that end in "skin": calfskin, lambskin, snakeskin, crocodile skin, and so on. For accessories (especially shoes), check the symbols present on the label. Faux leather is represented by a symbol that looks like a diamond, whereas real leather will look like a cowhide.

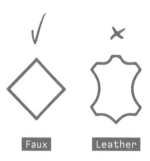

Faux   Leather

FUR

Mink, muskrat, fox, sable, beaver, karakul, raccoon, mole, marten, weasel, rabbit, coney, rex, lapin, seal, astrakhan, chinchilla, ermine.

WOOL

Merino, vicuña, angora, cashmere, alpaca, llama, mohair.

Other non-vegan words to look out for:
Silk, down, feathers, bones, horns, teeth (yes, there is jewelry that contains animal teeth, believe it or not).

VEGAN STYLE

DOS AND DON'TS
for creating a capsule wardrobe

do...
EVALUATE YOUR LIFESTYLE

Just saying, it might not be very useful to build your base around ripped jeans and biker boots if your job requires you to wear a power suit on a daily basis. Take a look at your life and what clothing might work for the majority of your needs.

~~~

DRESS FOR YOUR BODY SHAPE

It doesn't matter if everyone and their grandma claims that pencil skirts are the best skirt shape in the history of perfectly fitting jersey—if they don't suit your shape, you're never going to love them. If your figure is flattered by full skirts instead, go for it.

~~~

don't...
PLAY BY THE NUMBERS

I've seen some bloggers and style journalists say "pick a number, such as twenty items, and stick to it." I don't agree. For simplicity's sake, I list ten items in this chapter that, together, make up a great capsule wardrobe, but don't get hung up on the number itself—if you only need seven, choose seven. It's not the number of things that counts but how versatile each item is.

~~~

LIMIT YOURSELF

So you're curvy but love horizontal stripes? Or flat-chested but adore dramatic V-necks? *Big deal.* If you're happy in it, I say wear it. Simple as that. After all, there's a reason why you love this particular style, meaning that you'll probably look great in it. As long as you love it on *you*, not just on Kate Moss (the mirror is your best friend here).

BE CLIMATE CONSCIOUS

And I'm not just talking "climate" in the eco sense—more literally, don't disregard your local weather conditions. As much as I'd love for light denim jackets and breezy sandals to be part of my capsule wardrobe, I live in the United Kingdom, and, most of the time, the weather demands boots and thick knits. Any clothing that's too summer-specific will spend most of the year in my closet.

FASHION

THE TOP TEN ITEMS
for your capsule wardrobe

You can craft your capsule wardrobe to suit your needs, but there are a few essentials that no one should be without.

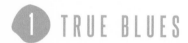 **TRUE BLUES**

I want you to do something for me. Go to your closet right now and open it. Count the pairs of jeans it contains, and you'll quickly realize the power of this omnipresent wardrobe classic (chances are, you're wearing a pair). At least one pair of jeans, often many more, is the backbone of any wardrobe, be it a woman's or a man's. Offering an endless supply of styles, washes, and cuts, jeans are the ultimate style staple.

Invented in 1871 by Latvian-American tailor Jacob Davis in partnership with Levi Strauss, jeans were originally designed for cowboys and miners, but evolved to become a trend essential in the 1950s. Excellent resistance and durability made denim a favorite among the casual crowd and the style set alike, with some of the most well-known icons being James Dean in *Rebel Without a Cause* and Debbie

Harry, who was one of the first fashionistas to introduce the double-denim look. And who can forget Farrah Fawcett's fitted flares, or the cast of *Beverly Hills, 90210* in their jeans?

Our true blues have come a long way since Levi's 501s ruled our wardrobes: there is no longer just one key style of the season. Today, a variety of cuts, from body-tight skinnies to nonchalant, relaxed boyfriend designs, are readily available to denim lovers. Personally, I favor a dark-washed flare, due to its power to make my legs look like they belong on a Victoria's Secret catwalk (no easy feat, believe me), but dark skinnies and distressed denim will also always have a place in my wardrobe. You should aim to build your jeans collection around your needs and lifestyle—how much will you be wearing them, when, where, and with what?

Four reasons to love jeans

1

They're the ultimate day-to-night piece. Add a floaty, feminine blouse to your dark-washed skinnies or flares, and this style staple will take you effortlessly from office to cocktails.

2

They're chic *and* comfortable. Well-fitting jeans won't squeeze, scratch, or hang around your knees. The stretch component in denim means that they fit snugly yet softly, making them the perfect blend of comfort and elegance.

Vegan jeans by Monkee Genes

3

They last forever. Hands up if you've still got your high school jeans (bonus points if they're pastel-colored). High resistance is one of the winning points of this evergreen item. Bonus: if you happen to rip your jeans, just add a few more rips, and voilà—a "distressed" style.

4

The endless supply of choice. Dark today, light tomorrow. Boyfriend style by day, sexy skinnies by night. Flared for the office, ripped for the weekend. You name it, there's a denim style for it.

SANDBLASTING

Most jeans, if not all, are vegan-friendly. The main fabric is cotton, so animals are rarely harmed in the making of denim. But, in some cases, there are still hazards connected to the manufacturing process—and one of these is sandblasting.

Sandblasting is one of the most talked-about side effects of denim production. It's used to give jeans that "worn" look. Sandblasting, carried out by factory workers, is done with a hose, an air compressor, and sand, so what it does is literally blast the fabric with sand, creating a faded effect.

Why is sandblasting an issue? When silica dust particles from the sand enter workers' lungs, they can create a condition called silicosis, which causes shortness of breath and coughing. If left untreated, silicosis can be fatal.

Both Levi's and H&M have banned sandblasting in their factories. After multiple cases of workers coming down with severe illnesses and several deaths from silicosis, Turkey issued a ban on manual sandblasting with silica in garment factories, which was a huge step forward, since Turkey is one of the world's largest denim exporters. But many industry insiders claim that sandblasting just moved to other territories (most of them in Asia).

BRANDS THAT ARE GOOD TO THE EARTH AND YOUR BODY

If you're outraged by the previous paragraph, fret not; you don't have to forgo your denim addiction. Just remember to do your research when shopping for jeans—how was your pair made, where, and by whom? For example, if you look out for the Global Organic Textile Standard (GOTS) certification, you can be sure that the garment you're buying is protected by a standard that prohibits sandblasting. It also ensures that the garment is made with 95 percent organic materials.

Nudie Jeans

The brand's 2006 goal of 100 percent organic production paid off—today, every pair is indeed organic. Nudie Jeans is also big on transparency, sharing its production guidelines with its customers, meaning you can follow the journey of your jeans and see where your pair was made.

Monkee Genes

"No blood, no sweat, no tears" is part of the brand's motto. Boasting certifications by the Soil Association and the GOTS, Monkee has also supported the Save the Bees campaign in the United Kingdom. Plus, they're PETA-approved vegan.

Levi's

The iconic denim label made the switch to eco-friendly in 2011, when it started crafting jeans made with cotton from the Better Cotton Initiative, a scheme that promotes sustainable cotton production.

Kuyichi

Working with organic cotton, recycled PET, and other eco-fabrics such as Tencel (sustainably produced Lyocell fibers), this Dutch brand also guarantees that your denim is free from child labor and slavery.

② THE WEAR-IT-EVERYWHERE DRESS

Dresses are a key staple because of their irresistible versatility. Whether it's a structured daytime shift, a laid-back denim dress for the weekend, or an evening sheath (or possibly all three), a dress is probably the most wearable piece in your wardrobe. A dress has the power to be effortless, sophisticated, and instantly chic—and it smoothly removes the "what top to wear with what bottom" dilemma.

Not really a dress person? You can easily swap this one out for a jumpsuit. A glamorous 1970s Halston-inspired design is sleek and versatile, while a utility-chic denim number says laid-back casual like nothing else. Jumpsuits are perhaps the easiest garment of all, providing a one-stop outfit solution that requires no further planning, and they effortlessly stand out from the crowd. Few items in my wardrobe are as commented on or complimented as the black, wrap-style, short-sleeved, wide-leg jumpsuit that I've owned for almost five years.

NOT JUST AN LBD

Notice that nowhere in this chapter have I written the words "little black" before "dress." I'm not just talking about one specific type of dress, as black dresses may not be hits with all women. I've noticed a takeover of black on the streets of most cities I've lived in during the last few years, one I definitely consider myself a part of, and who can blame us? Black is versatile, it's easy to match, and it instantly pulls your look together. But do a little research on how women dress in certain parts of South America or some parts of Asia, and our penchant for (or should I say obsession with) black all of a sudden seems bleak and conformist. I think stepping away from black and introducing even the subtlest hint of hue into your wardrobe can be liberating. All of a sudden, you find that you *do* look good in color, that you *can* wear prints, and that you're not necessarily confined to a monochromatic life.

Your capsule wardrobe dress can be black, but it might also be red, blue, green, pink, striped, printed, or whatever you prefer. As long as it's a dress you can see yourself wearing over and over again, matching it with a variety of items in your wardrobe, working in a number of seasons and making you feel like a million bucks every time you wear it, go for it. Even if it's really, really bright.

Here are some labels that provide vegan-friendly dresses

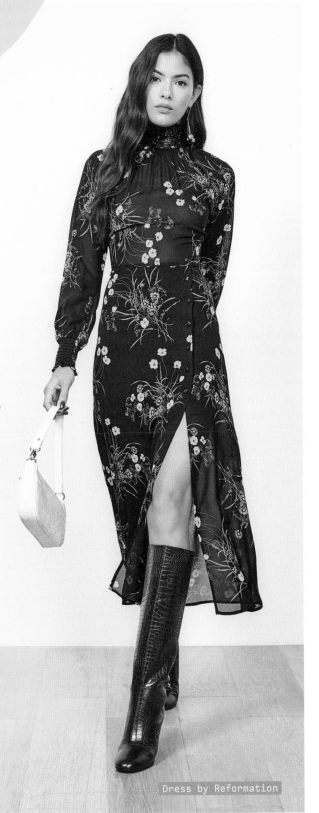

- **People Tree**

  The pioneers of fair-trade fashion, People Tree was founded by eco-entrepreneur Safia Minney. Using only natural dyes, People Tree is famous for feminine dresses in organic fabrics.

- **Free People**

  The ultimate in hippie chic, Urban Outfitters' boho-inflected sister brand Free People is rich in vegan options, including "leather" jackets and bags. But it's their dresses that win our hearts, thanks to their romantic, free-spirited feel.

- **Reformation**

  Sustainable style doesn't get any cooler than this. This Los Angeles label crafts most of its designs in its own sustainable sewing factory. The brand uses renewable energy and 100 percent recycled packaging. They also launch eco-themed capsule collections such as "Low Carb"— that's low CO_2 footprint—for events like Earth Day.

Dress by Reformation

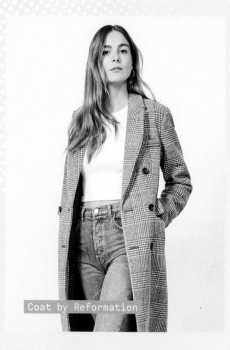

Coat by Reformation

Every year, when the days get shorter and temperatures drop, the dilemma of what to wear takes on a new, more complicated guise: your winter coat is doubtlessly the item of clothing that will work the hardest during the winter months, meaning it needs more than a little thought.

Finding a well-fitting, non-bulky winter coat with no wool is the vegan equivalent of winning the lottery (and I'm talking big-bucks win here). Wool is considered the universal warming material: without it, no winterwear can exist, apparently. And if it does, it's often dyed a garish color and will make you look like you're ten pounds heavier than you are, with mysterious lumps around your waist where the material bunches up when you walk, sit, breathe, or do anything at all. In my first winter season as a vegan, I often found myself staring wistfully at sleekly clad women on the train, wrapped up in soft throws, oversized ponchos, and sleek, structured coats, wishing to find even a smidgen of that kind of variety in the ranges suitable for vegans.

WHAT'S WRONG WITH WEARING WOOL?

One of the most common questions I get as a vegan, and especially as a lover of vegan fashion, is "What's wrong with wearing wool?" The answer is: A lot. Sheep are often kept in cramped spaces, and lambs' tails are cut off and their ears are hole-punched at just a few weeks old. Furthermore, the shearing process is far from "pleasurable" for sheep, despite what many wool brands might have us believe. As workers are often paid by the quantity of wool, not by the hour, they work quickly, frequently cutting and nicking the animals and, in some cases, even leaving wounded or sick animals with no veterinary care. See PETA's investigations into the wool industry at investigations.peta.org/australian-wool-industry-cruelty and check out chapter 9 of this book (page 212) for more on wool. Oh, and one more important detail: sheep do not need to be shorn. In nature, they grow just enough wool to protect themselves from the elements, whereas the wool industry deliberately breeds them to produce much more wool than they would do naturally—sometimes they can hardly stand up because of the excess weight.

WINTER WARMERS WITH A CONSCIENCE

VAUTE is a New York City brand founded by designer Leanne Mai-ly Hilgart. An animal-rights activist since childhood, Leanne creates beautiful, well-made, quality coats from recycled and recyclable vegan-friendly materials. After becoming the first 100 percent vegan brand to show at New York Fashion Week, VAUTE is the go-to brand for ethically produced vegan coats.

What's mulesing?

The practice of "mulesing" is particularly gruesome. Most of the world's wool comes from Australia, and the merino sheep being bred for wool there are sometimes subjected to this practice, which is particularly painful and uncomfortable, and can pose a real threat to the sheep's lives. As sheep have been bred to produce more wool than they would naturally need, a condition called flystrike can develop, in which flies lay eggs in the folds of the sheep's skin—eggs from which maggots are born that can literally eat the sheep alive. In an attempt to stop flystrike, farmers who practice mulesing cut off pieces of the sheep's skin to eliminate surplus folds where flies can lay eggs. This can lead to infections, which have caused many mulesed sheep to suffer and even die. A large variety of companies such as Hugo Boss, Adidas, H&M, and many more are very mindful that their wool not come from mulesed sheep, and mulesing is also banned in New Zealand.

MANUEL ORTIZ

CO-CREATOR OF WOOCOA

"Our intent is to legalize the labor and knowledge of former marijuana growers to grow hemp."

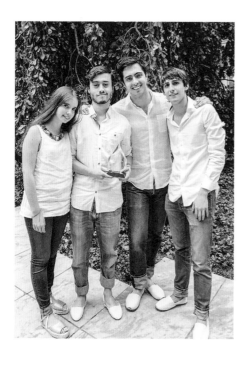

Students at Colombian Universidad de los Andes are the brains behind the latest eco-friendly material.

〰

A team of students at the Colombian Universidad de los Andes in Bogotá have crafted Woocoa, a wool-like product that is made from hemp, mushroom enzymes, and coconut fibers. For their innovative product, students Ana Laura Andrade, Iván Caballero, Moises Hernández, and Manuel Ortiz, under the direction of Giovanna Danies and Luz Alba Gallo, and with collaboration by Carolina Obregón and Johann Osma, were awarded the top prize in the PETA 2018 Biodesign Challenge to find the best new vegan-friendly material.

So what exactly is Woocoa, and how is it made? Manuel Ortiz, one of the creators of the material, explains:

Woocoa is a
blend of
coconut and
hemp fibers.

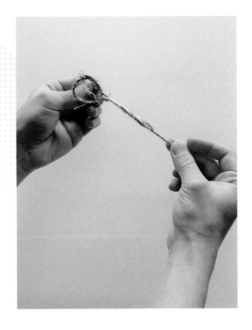

We first settled on using coconut fibers based on a previous project to replicate "coco-form," a material made with coconut and natural latex to make biodegradable packaging with thermal insulation. With this, we were able to emulate the hygroscopic properties of wool, which is able to wick humidity and maintain heat. Then, we decided to blend this fiber with hemp fibers. As you may know, the fibers extracted from hemp were widely used in ancient times and are still used today to make a wide array of products. But the war on drugs completely eradicated its use for quite some time. Hemp is very durable, soft, breathable, and fine. We wished for Woocoa to be a noble material—that's why the extraction and production of these fibers will be handled by communities in the Caribbean region (who grow coconut and extract its fibers) and former illicit marijuana growers who used to work for drug cartels and the FARC guerrilla group.

The latter is an interesting case, since these people were forced into growing these kinds of crops, but with the peace deal signed in 2016, they were widely left without jobs. Our intent is to legalize their labor and knowledge in order to grow hemp.

The next challenge was very clear: hemp and coconut fibers clearly do not feel like wool, so we had to develop a way to make them softer and finer without losing their strength. Through our research, we found that we could use certain types of "white rot" fungi to lightly degrade the fibers, making them softer without using harmful chemicals. That way, we kept our promise to make the product environmentally sustainable.

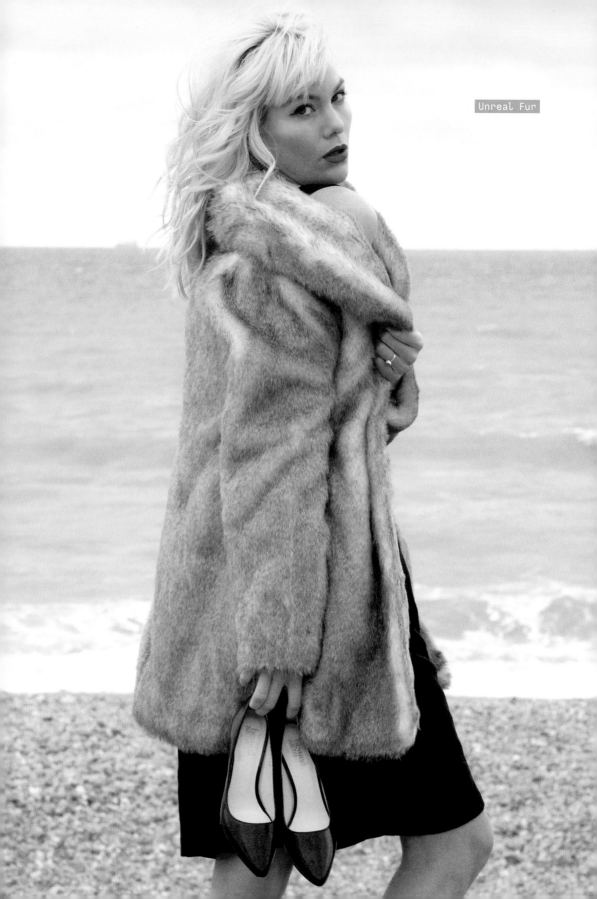

UNREAL FUR: THE AUSTRALIAN BRAND FOR THOSE WHO LOVE THE LOOK OF FUR, MINUS THE CRUELTY

You might not have been aware of the dark side of the wool industry, but you might know that 80 percent of all animals used for fur come from factory farms, where they are often held in small wire cages and deprived of pretty much all their natural behaviors, and the most common ways to kill them include gassing and poisoning. Conditions such as cannibalism and mutilation are not uncommon on fur factory farms. Animals who are trapped in the wild aren't much luckier, and are sometimes left in agony in traps for days until the trapper arrives and kills them. Some animals have been known to try to chew off their own limbs in an effort to escape.

Reading this and feeling guilty because you love the look of fur? No worries: Australian faux-fur brand Unreal Fur has you covered (quite literally). Offering a range of faux-fur garments that come in colors so natural that they look every bit like the real deal, or more out-there hues such as emerald green or deep burgundy, this brand has everything from coats and jackets to stylish faux-fur scarves. Faking it has never looked this good.

Other brands that fake it well

Ainea

This Italian brand isn't purely focused on fur, but offers some beautiful faux-fur coats and jackets.

Shrimps

Designer Hannah Weiland created this faux-fur brand that has become a darling of the London Fashion Week set. If you like colorful, standout coats, Shrimps will become your new obsession.

Jakke

A British brand offering a range of statement outerwear in faux fur for the trend-loving vegan. With faux furs in patterns such as checks or snake print, as well as attention-grabbing colors, this is a range for those who want to stand out from the crowd.

La Seine et Moi

French-girl chic with a vegan twist. This brand, awarded Best Vegan Fur by PETA, creates a collection of elegant, versatile faux-fur coats and jackets, complemented by a collection of bags with faux-fur detailing.

4 THE SKYSCRAPER HEELS

No capsule wardrobe is complete without The Heels—even Marilyn Monroe, who hardly needed any help in the seduction department, relied on heels to boost her appeal. "I don't know who invented high heels, but women owe him a lot" is one of her most famous quotes. And Marilyn was right: the heel, originating in medieval times and initially worn by men to obtain height and status, has become synonymous with femininity. Even if you're more of a flats person, you probably have at least one pair of fabulous heels in your wardrobe. Few things have the power to transform your look the way a pair of heels can—not only do they add a few inches, they also streamline your silhouette and even alter your walk. There is no evening dress that isn't beautifully set off with the right pair of heels, be it a playful cocktail number or a spectacular gala gown. Forget diamonds—heels are a girl's best friend.

It's a common misconception that high heels, or any shoes for that matter, have to be made of leather to be good-quality and/or in style. Brands like Free People and Marais USA are incorporating vegan styles into their selections for a reason—they recognize the trend, and the're not about to skimp on quality.

Where to shop for cruelty-free heels

Cult of Coquette
The sky-high, daring, unapologetic heel. Available in a myriad of hues—all cruelty-free.

Sydney Brown
Not all heels are created equal. Maybe your capsule-wardrobe heel is a wedge—in which case you'll love this Los Angeles shoe designer's eco-friendly styles. I'm also a fan of their curved-heel pumps.

Bourgeois Boheme
Colorful and flirty, these are the ultimate day-to-night heels. This British brand produces their styles in Portugal, using eco-friendly, PVC-free materials.

Olsenhaus
Designer Elizabeth Olsen crafts edgy footwear that's as haute as any leather shoe you'll find stomping down the catwalks at Fashion Week, if not more so. Her sweatshop-free styles include ankle boots, pumps, and wedges.

HEATHER WHITTLE

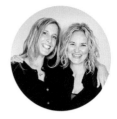

COFOUNDER OF BEYOND SKIN

"We're thrilled to be able to offer our customers design-driven, stylish, ethical shoes."

Heather (left)
and Natalie
(right)

〜〜

When it comes to heels, the fashionistas behind this Brighton-based vegan shoe brand know their stuff—their shoes have been worn by Natalie Portman, and Bond girl Olga Kurylenko even wore a pair of their heels to the Oscars. Those are some serious style credentials. Heather explains the values behind the brand:

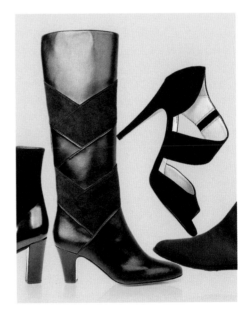

We personally shop for shoes by their design, closely followed by the quality of their materials, which is always a factor to take into consideration. We check what the shoes are made from and make sure no PVC is involved, or any other harmful substances. Where the shoes are produced is also crucial. These values are really important to us.

Our customer is seeking out a stylish shoe that's cruelty-free, and this customer is influenced by general fashion trends. They aspire to wear stylish footwear without sacrificing their ethics, and we're thrilled to be able to offer them a product with a very different aesthetic: vintage-inspired, design-driven, stylish, ethical shoes.

Creating a
chic and
functional
wardrobe that's
free from
animal-derived
fabrics has
never been
easier.

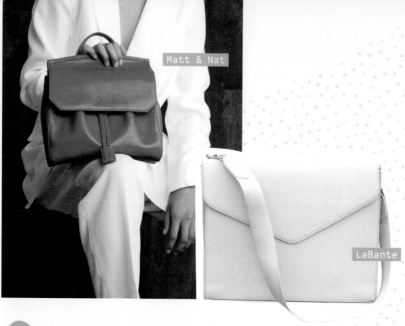

Matt & Nat

LaBante

5 THE DAYTIME BAG

The age-old adage that women "carry their world around in their bags" hits close to home. The daytime tote bag is an absolute must in the wardrobe of every woman, especially one who works full-time; the sheer amount of stuff we carry around on a daily basis is pretty crazy. Women only started to use bags in the nineteenth century—before that, they had detachable pouches on their petticoats. But, as fashions changed, pocket space was reduced and new solutions were born.

Today, bags have risen beyond simple functionality and become status symbols. If you look at the accessory selection of a designer fashion brand, the priciest items are often the bags. Due to their highly recognizable design, bags are often the most covetable pieces in a designer's collection. But another reason

that the price of the latest "It" bag soars above your monthly rent is the material—calfskin and lamb leather being among those considered most exclusive, while alligator and lizard skins add further zeros to the price tag. But look beyond the heavyweight fashion labels and you'll be surprised at what you'll find: faux leather has never looked so good, and compassionate fashionistas know it.

The first designer to introduce faux to international catwalks, Stella McCartney is responsible for every vegan shopaholic's dream bag: the Falabella. Available in a variety of colors and sizes, this sleek tote flies in the face of the hemp-sack stereotype; it's contemporary and chic, just like the conscious shoppers who carry it.

Vegan "It" bags: the ultimate wish list

Stella McCartney

The ultimate vegan dream bag. The number-one sign that you've "made it" for a vegan isn't a Gucci bag or Manolo Blahnik heels, it's a Falabella from Queen Stella on our arm.

Jill Milan

When you've got Jennifer Lawrence, Anne Hathaway, and Eva Longoria carrying your glamorous clutches and chic shoulder bags, you know that vegan fashion is here to stay.

LaBante London

On seeing the refined designs from LaBante London, you wouldn't expect them to be made with recycled materials. But that is indeed the truth: each bag is lined with recycled fabrics.

Matt & Nat

This Canadian brand has become somewhat of a classic in the vegan world, and for good reason: creating men's and women's bags in subdued, sophisticated hues, this brand has made it to the top of every vegan wish list. Bonus: the linings of their bags are made from recycled plastic bottles.

Angela Roi

If you're looking for something truly luxurious, go for an elegant design from this US brand, which donates part of its proceeds to animal charities. Looking good and doing good—that's the way of the modern vegan.

6 THE AUTUMN-WINTER KNIT

And so we enter tricky territory. As materials and technology advance, winterwear for vegans is slowly emerging, but pickings are still relatively slim. Since manufacturing processes are largely kept under wraps, wool is still regarded as a relatively harmless product. The process of mulesing (see page 31) is still relatively unknown, and people still associate wool with happy, fluffy lambs rather than filthy cages and blood. But times are changing, and if I had trouble finding a knit without that 8 percent wool when I was starting my journey as a vegan shopper, these days it's much easier.

Through the chillier months, nothing is as versatile as the right knit. Paired with your jeans (see page 24) or a midi skirt, it's the perfect mix of cozy and chic. For the weekend, dress it down with a miniskirt or skinny trousers. Throw on your coat or your "leather" jacket (see page 48) and you're good to go.

While I might not always agree with American Apparel's advertising policies (remember that website imagery where a tartan "unisex" shirt was worn by a normally dressed male model . . . and then a female model sans underwear? Yeah, I think many of us do with

disgust), this brand does cater to vegan shoppers with a selection of wool-free knits. Mostly cotton with a hint of acrylic, American Apparel's slouchy styles are an easy way to stay on-trend while eschewing wool.

San Francisco–based eco label Everlane is worth checking out for more than knits. Placing emphasis on transparency, Everlane encourages their customer to "always ask why," constantly challenging the status quo. Their website offers extensive info on their factories around the world, making it possible for people to research how the clothing is made. Everlane doesn't outsource or overproduce, sticking to the basics to create simple, wearable separates for everyday life. If it's breezy, early-spring knits you're after, you're in luck; their super-soft French Terry knits are completely vegan and represent the ultimate in comfort and laid-back style. Just watch out for the merino wool, which appears in some of their designs.

British brand White Stuff is also a hero for knit-loving vegans, offering chic cardigans and off-duty sweaters in muted tones, or decorated with playful prints. Once again, this isn't a vegan brand but one that offers vegan-friendly designs, so keep an eye on the labels.

The year-round knit

Not just for cold weather, the ultimate knit (not too heavy, not too flimsy) can earn its place in your capsule wardrobe due to its versatility. Here's how to wear it all year.

WINTER

▽

This one's easy. Pair your knit with slim, black trousers tucked into boots—whether you dare to go knee-high, opt for the rock-chic look with biker boots, or add a bit of height with ankle boots. All you need to add is your capsule-wardrobe coat, and your perfect winter look is complete.

SPRING

◁

Throw on your sweater over distressed jeans and Converse sneakers, topping it off with a colorful statement bag for a look that adapts well to unpredictable weather.

SUMMER

▽

If, like me, you live in a country where tropical weather isn't guaranteed even in the warmer months (I love you for many reasons, Britain, but weather isn't one of them), then you can layer up by pairing a light knit with a miniskirt to leave your legs bare, complementing the look with dainty flats or chunky-heeled sandals.

AUTUMN

▽

When the first chills of the year arrive, style your trusty knit with a shirt dress, tights, and ankle boots for an outfit that exudes nonchalant cool.

FASHION

⑦ THE CLASSIC T-SHIRT

A true wardrobe must, the T-shirt is at the core of the capsule wardrobe. So many outfits can be built around it, from a relaxed summer pairing with a floaty maxi skirt to urban styling with skinny jeans and boots. Jeans and T-shirts should form the backbone of your capsule wardrobe, simply because they will take you through so many everyday occasions. The right T-shirt is the perfect blend of slouchy and structured—not too loose-fitting, but never tight. The trick is in the fit: I sometimes try on twenty T-shirts before I find the one that fits just right.

I usually go for a round neck over a V-neck, but that really depends on what looks better on you. What's important to keep in mind when scrutinizing a potential purchase in the dressing-room mirror is the fit on the shoulders, the fall of the hem on the hips, and the cut—is it baggy? Is it too tight? Until you hit just the right cut, don't whip out your wallet.

The issue with cotton

Like jeans, T-shirts are often made from cotton, making the majority of them vegan. But the eco-minded among you should pay attention to a few matters, and the supply chain is one of them. Cotton production has a history of slavery, and many workers today are still paid way below minimum wage. India and Uzbekistan represent two of the world's most prominent cotton producers, and industries in both these countries have histories of child labor and extreme conditions. Safety is rarely a concern in some of the world's worst-off cotton factories, and teenagers are often left picking cotton in the fields late into the night.

Furthermore, cotton production is an environmental issue. Unless it's organic, cotton is often treated with fungicides and/or insecticides and heavily sprayed with pesticides, which can be toxic to humans and animals alike. These chemicals pollute soil and waterways, sometimes leaving a long-term footprint on the land where the cotton is grown. The solution? Look for organic cotton, which is significantly better when it comes to these issues.

VEGAN STYLE

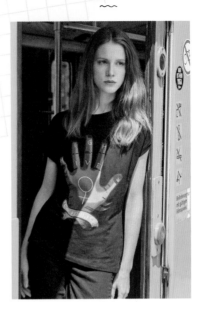

Morning to midnight: A day in the life of the perfect T-shirt

7:30 am

WAKE-UP CALL

Styled with slim trousers
and a well-cut blazer.
Topped off with ankle
boots and a roomy daytime
bag for the office.

1 pm

LUNCHTIME

Throw on a printed faux-silk
scarf and sunglasses for
laid-back chic.

5:30 pm

HAPPY HOUR!

A sequined skirt and peep-toe
boots do the trick, taking the
tee from day to dusk.

7 pm

DINNER

Add a high-glamour sheen
with a statement necklace
and a fitted jacket.

A quick note on nuance . . .

You'll notice that "white" isn't
mentioned anywhere near "T-shirt."
As discussed with the little black
dress, color is entirely up to you.
Maybe your perfect T-shirt is white,
or maybe it's bright. Mine is black.
But a good rule of thumb here,
unlike with dresses, is to stick
to laid-back, neutral hues. Your
capsule wardrobe tee might not
be white, but it's unlikely to be a
neon color, either; make those
playful extras and leave your
capsule collection for basics in
gray, black, taupe, khaki, and—
you guessed it—white.

8 THE EVENING CLUTCH

You'll notice that up until now, we've been talking daywear, or, in some cases, day-to-night wear, as I like to call it. That's because the winning feature of most capsule items is versatility—they look just as effortless by day as they do by night. Our first exception: the clutch.

The clutch is pure evening finery. Whether it's sleek and minimalist or lavishly embellished, this accessory never sees the light of day—unless you're from my home country of Sweden, where summer nights remain light until almost midnight. You get my point: the clutch is not a daytime bag. This is proved by its dramatically tiny proportions—most clutches are just barely big enough to fit a credit card and a lipstick. This accessory is more of a showpiece, a style detail, than an actual practicality; such is the way of the fashion world. And this is exactly why we eschew restraint and pull out all the stops with sequins, beads, and metallics. Clutches are the silver lining of the capsule wardrobe.

WILBY: MASTERS OF THE VEGAN CLUTCH

Most handbag brands are born from a desire to create practical daytime bags, with clutches as a complementary extra, but this is not true of all brands.

British brand Wilby has clutches at its core. Launched in 2013 in London, Wilby specializes in faux-leather clutches using eco-materials such as organic cotton and cork leather. Their sleek collections have now branched out into bigger bags as well, all carrying the PETA-approved vegan trademark. Perfect for injecting color into your capsule wardrobe without going overboard on decoration, these bags provide an ample range of any-occasion accessories: pair the Drayton with a structured bodycon dress, or go for a bright Primrose clutch to liven up a laid-back LBD. The options are endless.

The many faces of the clutch

Few accessories have as much change-it-up potential as the clutch: its many guises offer endless possibilities.

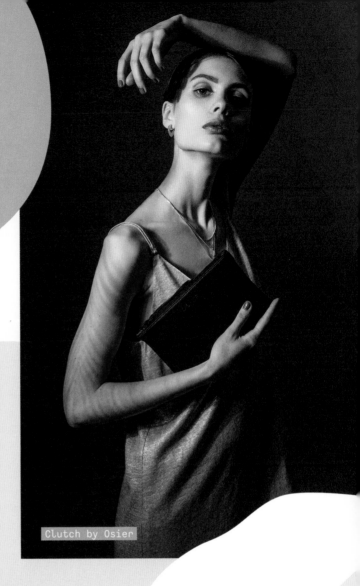

Clutch by Osier

THE BOXY CLUTCH

Maybe the roomiest of them all. Sturdy and versatile, this clutch can offer a futuristic finish or a vintage feel.

THE ENVELOPE CLUTCH

Not good for carrying more than the aforementioned credit card and lipstick. Even when oversized, the envelope clutch looks best when almost empty.

THE WRISTLET CLUTCH

Elegant, refined, and playful. But don't be fooled—there's still hand-holding to do.

THE CHAIN CLUTCH

The comfortable fashionista's choice. Can't be bothered to hold anything while dancing? Just sling the chain strap over your shoulder and whirl away.

9 THE (NON) LEATHER JACKET

This is perhaps the most versatile item in your capsule collection. The perfect faux-leather jacket, once you find it, will accompany you from morning to evening, from the office to cocktails, and, last but definitely not least, through those oh-so-annoying in-between seasons when you're neither warm nor cold. It will masterfully top off your perfect jeans as well as virtually any dress, and add that elusive hint of cool, slightly rebellious nonchalance. In other words, it's a must.

Why not leather?

Leather is a coproduct of the meat industry. It's reductive to claim that leather exists just because the skins of animals used for meat would be "wasted" otherwise. This is simply not the case. The two industries mutually lean on each other, and one wouldn't be as profitable without the other. Over 1 billion animals die for the leather trade every year, including cows, calves, lambs, and goats, but also, shockingly, dogs and cats. China is among the world's biggest leather exporters, and, due to a complete lack of animal welfare laws, it's not unusual for Chinese leather producers to utilize the furry friends we know as our pets and family members (see page 61).

Despite what the leather industry would have you believe, leather is far from environmentally friendly. Water depletion and air and water pollution are just a few of the issues connected to this cruel trade. And don't believe the hype around "vegetable-dyed" leather either; keeping animals for leather is a waste of precious environmental resources long before the animal is killed and any dyeing/tanning takes place. Cruelty-free is the only truly ethical, environmentally sound choice.

The three golden rules of (non) leather jacket shopping

Make sure it's not too short. Even the biker variety shouldn't be super-short, so don't forget to look at how it falls in the back to avoid a 1980s-throwback look (unless that's what you're going for).

Try to gauge whether the material will crack. This isn't easy, but, as a rule of thumb, if it's even a tiny bit creased already, chances are it will crack pretty quickly. Try to get a feel for how sturdy the material is—it should be soft yet thick and butter-smooth. If it feels flimsy or has creases, leave it on the rack.

Don't bother about how it will look zipped up. Because when are you ever going to zip it up? A leather jacket should be tossed over your outfit, not meticulously done up.

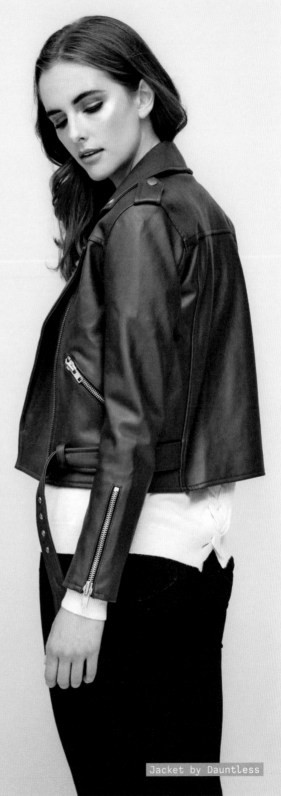

Jacket by Dauntless

I can't believe it's not leather: makers of the perfect vegan biker jackets

Dauntless

If you were a lover of leather jackets in your pre-vegan life (and I sure was), you will fall head over heels for Dauntless, a US-based brand specializing in—yep, you guessed it—vegan biker jackets, lined with faux silk. Whether you prefer traditional black or unusual shades like bright red or pale pink, it's likely you'll find your new favorite jacket at Dauntless.

Blank NYC

An edgy New York brand that focuses on jeans, this urban label also carries faux-leather jackets, trousers, and skirts in high-quality vegan leather. Not all their designs are vegan, so check the label before you buy.

Ovide

This French eco-friendly brand offers biker jackets in . . . cork! If you want to be truly innovative and support the use of reusable, recyclable materials (I could write a whole book on the wonders of cork), try an Ovide jacket.

Cornelia Guest with Project Gravitas

Cornelia Guest is probably one of the people I'd invite to my fantasy dinner party, just to hear all her stories. This is a woman who's done it all and more. She's been on the cover of *Time* magazine (topless), been named Debutante of the Decade in 1986, had Andy Warhol as a guest at her eighteenth birthday party, and was close friends with Truman Capote. She's also done an "I'd Rather Go Naked than Wear Fur" campaign for PETA, published a vegan cookbook, and designed a line of cruelty-free handbags. To top it all off, she designed a line of faux-leather biker jackets for Project Gravitas. The three styles—Nelson, Olive, and Lyle—carried an air of nonchalant cool, though for a variety of reasons are virtually impossible to buy now.

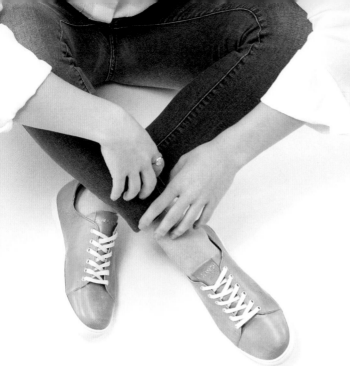

Unexpected ways to wear your sneakers

Pair them with a pleated midi skirt.

~~~

Break off a sequined minidress with white Converse.

~~~

Give tailored trousers a rebellious streak with black or studded sneakers.

~~~

Liven up an all-black look with a neon pair.

~~~

Team a floral dress with lived-in Supergas or Vans.

10 THE WORK-TO-WEEKEND SNEAKERS

Last but definitely not least on the list is an item you probably already have a few of in your closet—the one you rely on for lazy Sunday walks and quick runs to the supermarket, as well as city weekend breaks with lots of landmarks to trot to and from. Yep, we're talking sneakers.

Once limited to workout territory, sneakers have taken the step from the gym to the catwalk. Photographers snapping street-style shots outside recent international fashion weeks probably never saw so many flat shoes, let alone sporty styles. With sports-luxe came the sports shoe, which is good news for cruelty-free fashionistas, as many sneaker styles are leather-free.

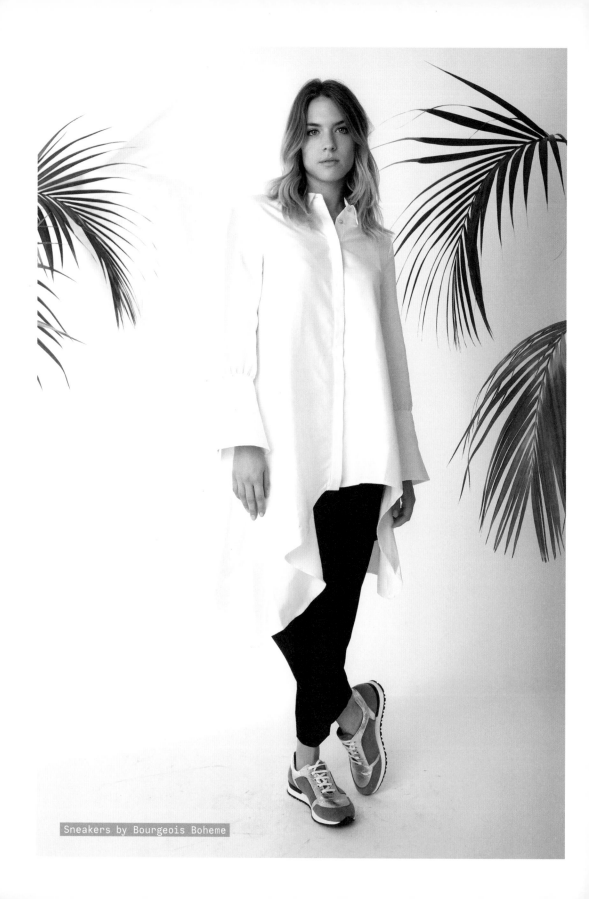

Sneakers by Bourgeois Boheme

ONCE AND FOR ALL: ARE CONVERSE VEGAN?

Their canvas-and-rubber exterior might have made them appear as the perfect cruelty-free option—and, in many cases, they are. But beware of what lurks beneath: in some pairs of Converse, it's animal glue.

A staffer on my magazine once wrote to Converse HQ asking for clarification—and their reply was that it differs from model to model. So there you have it; there is no "once and for all." If there's a specific pair you like, my advice is to contact the label and ask about that specific pair. The same goes for Supergas and Vans: some styles are vegan, others aren't. But then again—and some of you might not agree with me on this one—when you buy faux-leather shoes, some of them will have animal glue and you'll never know. So, while it's definitely a good idea to find out as much as possible and let brands know why you care about these issues, remember that, as vegans, we can't possibly be perfect, and traces of animal products are going to sneak in. So don't beat yourself up.

The age-old decision: high-top or low-top?

As someone who lives in high-top sneakers, you'd think I'd be biased. However, there's much to say for low-top styles: they're easier to match, they're sleeker and less bulky, and they offer more variety, while high-tops are more of a statement look and offer an urban finish.

WEAR HIGH-TOPS WITH

- Wide-leg, relaxed trousers.
- Straight, unstructured mini and midi skirts
- Rolled-up boyfriend jeans
- Tailored suits

WEAR LOW-TOPS WITH

- Skinny jeans
- Pleated skirts
- Maxi dresses
- A-line dresses and skirts

. . . but rules, as you know, are made to be broken.

ACCESS

ORIES

THE FINISHING TOUCHES

Think high-quality
accessories must be
made of leather?
Think again.

When I went vegetarian, giving up leather clothing and accessories was a given.

Coming to that conclusion was rather easy—I was desperate to do as much as I could for animals, so the thought of wearing their skins didn't appeal to me anymore. As I left leather behind, I couldn't help but notice—and be annoyed by—people's reverence for it, especially in the fashion industry. I heard people around me talking about "real leather" like it was something of value, something to show off—"this bag is real leather," which didn't sound like something to be proud of to me. As a teenager, I made a point of telling people that my shoes and bag *weren't* leather. But, back then, it was slim pickings: even the low-cost fashion chains where my entire wardrobe came from (this was before the dawn of sustainable style) strived to sell as many leather pieces as possible (always with the proud "Genuine Leather" label that I hated). If you chose to forgo animal skins, you were stuck with pleather—the shiny, plasticky kind that would crumble and rip after three wears. Heels of faux-leather shoes were also low-quality, and I spent a fortune on the maintenance of cheap shoes. Bags were almost always garish, brightly colored, and visibly low-quality.

Of course, even back in the day, there were people who were mindful of the waste of the mass-producing fashion chains. As an alternative, there was the odd eco shop, with its very limited fashion offerings—which were far from on-trend or luxurious. Heels were, of course, nowhere to be found. It annoyed me that the general idea seemed to be to choose between looking good and dressing compassionately.

Now I think back to those days and can't help but feel proud of how far we've come. Today, fashion magazines swoon over the Falabella, Stella McCartney's signature "It" bag—100 percent faux leather. Jill Milan crafts stunning daytime totes and evening clutches in Italy, while stars like Olga Kurylenko wear vegan shoes from Beyond Skin to the Oscars, BHAVA Studio makes shoes that any fashion blogger would be proud to wear, and Cult of Coquette is the champion of glamorous vegan heels. But how did this style revolution happen? And could it be too good to be true?

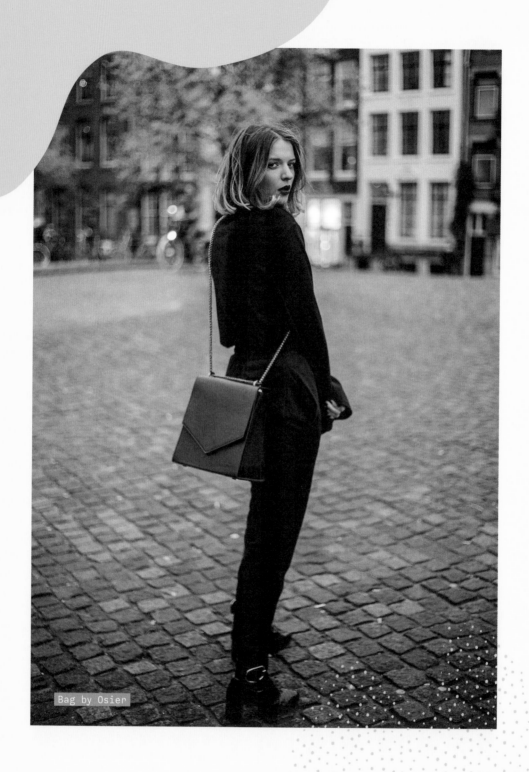

Bag by Osier

VEGAN STYLE

FAUX LEATHER
and the environment

Material-wise, faux leather has come a long way from the shiny, easy-to-crease "pleather" material of just a few years ago. Back then, vegan accessories were crafted from PVC—not exactly the environment's best friend, as it's not biodegradable—thus earning vegan leather a reputation as the opposite of eco. But these days, animal-free materials are a far cry from the PVC-laden pleather of the past.

Brands are investing time and resources in research, resulting in durable accessories that stand the test of time. Eco-minded designers such as Matt & Nat, who craft the linings of their fashionista-friendly bags from recycled plastic bottles, among other materials, set the bar high for eco-friendly designs, while shoe brand Bourgeois Boheme uses no PVC in its production processes, proving that the environmental argument against faux leather is slowly losing validity. Innovative brands are working on leather replacements made from pineapples, mushrooms, apples, and much more (see chapter 8, page 206, for more info on those).

In Italy, where I lived for six years, faux leather is referred to as "eco leather," and the same goes for faux fur—it's "eco fur." Recycled materials feature heavily in vegan fashion, further sustaining my argument that we as humans can work on our technologies to develop eco-friendly fabrics. The recent developments in high-tech synthetics and the repurposing of natural materials into leather-like fabrics show that the future isn't about optimizing leather—it's about perfecting animal-friendly fabrics.

CORK BAGS

the most ethical fashion accessories in the world?

Imagine a material that's 100 percent vegan, natural, renewable, and recyclable. This material is also flexible and durable at the same time, as well as water-resistant, and can easily be made into fashion accessories. Sounds like a dream, right? Well, wake up, because this miraculous material is already here, and you've probably seen it—but not on a bag. I'm talking about cork. Yes, cork, like in wine bottles. Turns out you can make bags from it, and they actually look good.

I know what you're thinking, but hear me out: you don't even have to cut down the cork trees to make cork bags—in fact, the cork oak tree from which it's harvested can live for around two hundred years. Portugal is rich in cork trees and enjoys a thriving cork industry, including so-called cork leather. Every nine years, the bark is separated from the tree without causing permanent damage, and it keeps growing back in a renewable cycle. Amazing, right? Well, that's not all: every time a cork oak tree is harvested, it absorbs extra carbon dioxide to aid the bark's regeneration process. Cork oak trees that are regularly harvested store three to five times more carbon dioxide than those left unharvested. Since only the bark is removed to obtain the cork, the tree goes on living and contributing to keeping the air clean.

So, we know that cork is environmentally amazing—but it's also durable, lightweight, easy to clean, and, surprisingly, really fashion-forward. In the last few years, bag brands specializing in cork have conquered the vegan fashion arena through attention to style and design. Just a decade ago, you probably wouldn't have thought of cork as fashionable, but thanks to brands realizing the appeal of looking good as well as doing good, cork is looking better than ever.

Cork brands to check out

- Nina Bernice
- Corkor
- Jentil Bags
- Rok Cork
- Corature

The horrifying truth behind China's dog and cat leather industry

Leather is a material that's very difficult to trace back to its origins. Your bag may say "made in France" or "made in the USA," but that only refers to where the bag was assembled, not where the actual leather came from. Of course, the "made in" factor helps raise a garment's or an accessory's status and therefore financial worth, but if consumers knew more about the materials that made up their exclusive accessory, chances are they wouldn't find it so appealing. If you try to trace the supply chain back to the actual animal, you'll find that it's very hard to uncover its true origins. And that's how dog leather accessories have ended up on the European market, sold to unwitting consumers.

China, where most of the world's fur and leather comes from—and where there are no laws to protect animals from abuse—has a large, thriving dog and cat leather industry that exports heavily. In 2014, a PETA Asia investigator visited a dog-leather factory and learned that this specific facility killed two to three hundred dogs per day, and their skins were sold all over the world. And, of course, they aren't labeled as "dog leather" in most places where they're sold, just as "leather." Chances are, unsuspecting consumers buy and wear these accessories without knowing (or questioning) where they come from. Check chapter 9 (page 212) for more tips on how to tell whether your leather (and fur) are really faux, and see the PETA investigation at investigations.peta.org/china-dog-leather (warning: it's really difficult viewing and very graphic footage).

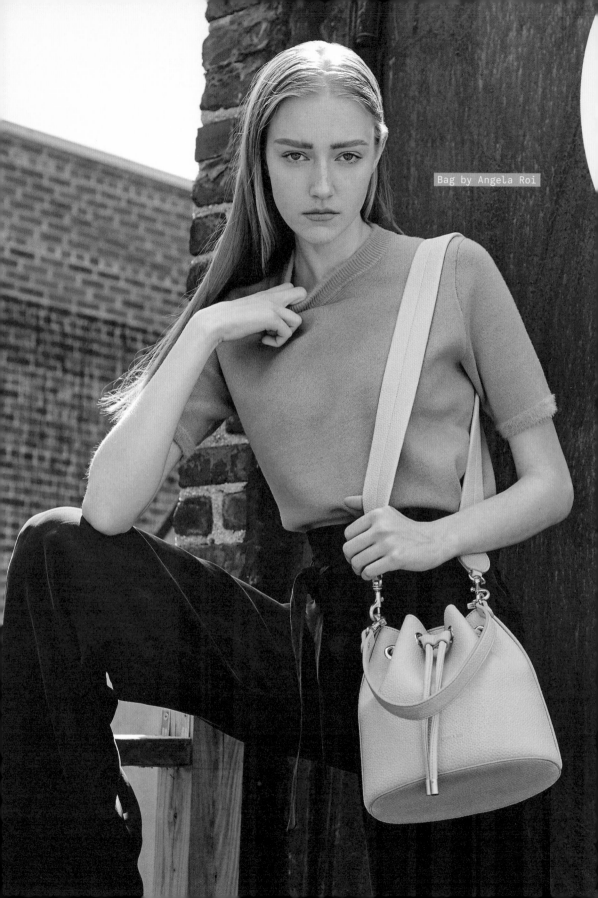
Bag by Angela Roi

BAGS, BAGS, BAGS
brand directory

Your collection of bags should be built according to your needs and lifestyle. As soon as you've got those figured out, check out these premium eco brands to make your picks.

DAYTIME

Angela Roi
The perfect work bags come courtesy of chic American brand Angela Roi. The ultimate in daytime sleek, these bags are made in a sweatshop-free factory in Korea. Minimalist yet attention-grabbing, Angela Roi bags come in a variety of colors and are spacious enough to fit everything you need for a day at work.

TRAVEL

Elvis & Kresse
Made from the most creative of recycled materials (decommissioned fire hose, anyone?), this brand donates part of its proceeds to the Fire Fighters Charity. The roomy travel bags are perfect for a weekend trip or as carry-on luggage—highly durable and truly unique, these are bags to keep forever. A word of warning: some of their bags have a silk lining, so, as usual, read the label.

SPECIAL OCCASIONS

Jill Milan
It's no wonder that celebs turn to Jill Milan for gala events—founders Jill Fraser and Milan Lazich have mastered the art of the after-dark accessory. Artful clutches and sophisticated minaudiéres set the brand apart from other faux-leather bag brands, most of whom specialize in daytime bags (Jill Milan's daytime bags are, by the way, amazing as well).

INNOVATIVE GLAMOUR

Alexandra K

This chic label from Poland uses eco-friendly materials like apple leather (see page 222) along with their own "Freedom Leather" (a sustainable, silicone-based vegan leather) to create high-end designer accessories that will make any vegan fashion lover reach for their wallet. Famous for their luxurious accessories, the brand also recently launched vegan biker jackets.

best for

VERSATILITY

Matt & Nat

What sets these bags apart isn't only their refined yet contemporary design but also their eco approach: Matt & Nat craft the linings of their bags from recycled bottles. Offering range after range of durable and elegant creations in easy-to-match, subdued shades, this is the go-to brand for versatile vegan accessories.

best for

INVESTMENT

Stella McCartney

The queen of eco-friendly runway hits, Stella's is the label that tempts even non-vegans to forgo leather. Rock royalty Stella has managed to do what few others could: break into mainstream fashion thanks to her clean and considered aesthetic. Investing in a Falabella is a classic case of "buy today, love forever," for Stella's designs are truly timeless and will accompany you through the years with never-ending grace.

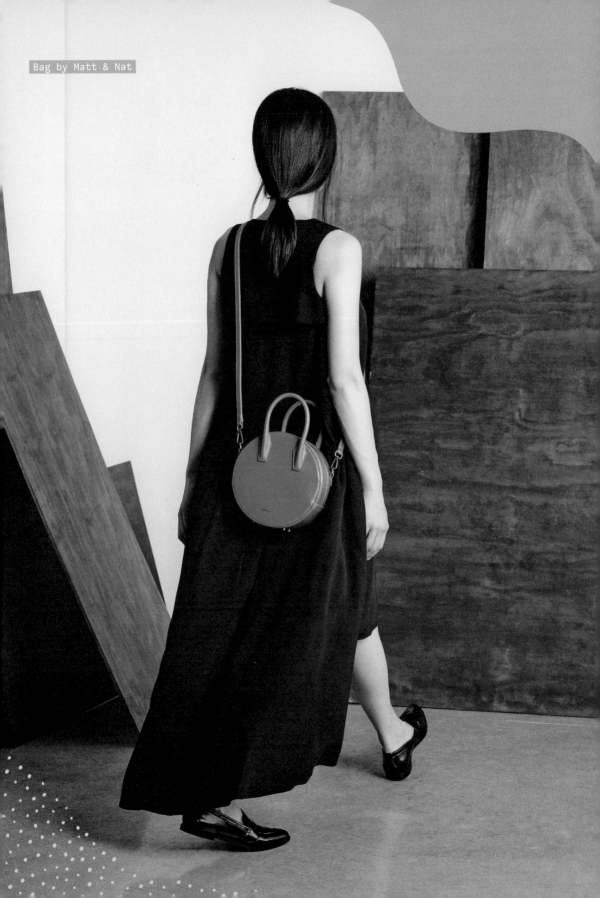

JILL FRASER

COFOUNDER OF JILL MILAN

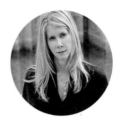

"Finding The One (bag, that is): it's all about individuality."

Jill Fraser and her partner, Milan Lazic, run the wildly successful vegan accessory brand Jill Milan (yep, those bags you've seen carried by Jennifer Lawrence, Kerry Washington, Eva Longoria, and more). Here's what Jill has to say about selecting the perfect bag:

To me, the key criteria for a must-have handbag is really what is most flattering for you. For instance, is the bag too small or too big? Is it too trendy or too conservative? These are all important factors to take into consideration when buying a bag. I often see women carrying bags that completely overwhelm them. It might be the "It" bag of the season, but it might look a lot better on a model than on the average person. Eva Longoria is extremely chic, and she often opts for clutches for daytime. Our clutches are big enough to carry a lot of items, and they never overwhelm the wearer. I wish more women would look at clutches for day.

Finally, I think a must-have bag should be durable and not be made through the exploitation of humans or animals. I'm vegan myself, and found it difficult to find vegan handbags that were also stylish and high in quality. I preferred a bag that I knew was made using fair-trade practices. I sensed there would be growing demand for such bags and decided to start a company myself to meet that demand. As a result, I've come to know a number of women who feel the way I do: they want animal-free fashion, but they also want it to be beautiful.

Our concepts are created by our designers, whose backgrounds include Prada, Judith Leiber, and other luxury brands. A skilled craftswoman with experience in construction creates the tech packs—the technical specifications for the atelier who will manufacture the bag. The designs and tech packs go on

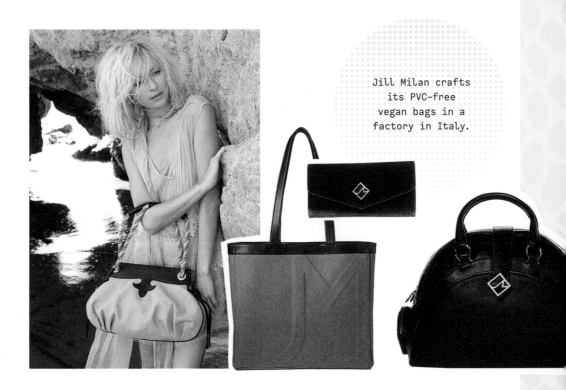

to the Italian manufacturer, and we begin reviewing fabric samples.

At this stage, I travel to Europe. Here, we meet with both the atelier and the metalworker. We commission first samples of any custom metalwork, while the artisans begin the process of cutting and sewing the first samples.

The first stage of the sampling process generally takes a few weeks, and we first see samples without metal and the final fabrics. At this stage, we typically make structural changes to the bags. For instance, do we think a strap should be lengthened? Should the bag be a bit shorter, longer, etc.?

During the second stage of the sampling process, we see the bags with the custom metal and with the fabrics we've selected for sampling. We narrow the samples now, selecting only the best fabrics.

Finally, we select fabrics, zippers, feet, and other supplies, and the atelier schedules the bags for production. In selecting these materials, we try to find fabrics that are durable and as eco-friendly as possible. Many leathers in China can be purchased for under $3, but we use fabrics with wholesale costs as high as $68 per yard. These materials are both beautiful and durable.

You can
succeed in
staying stylish
while keeping
your cruelty-
free values.

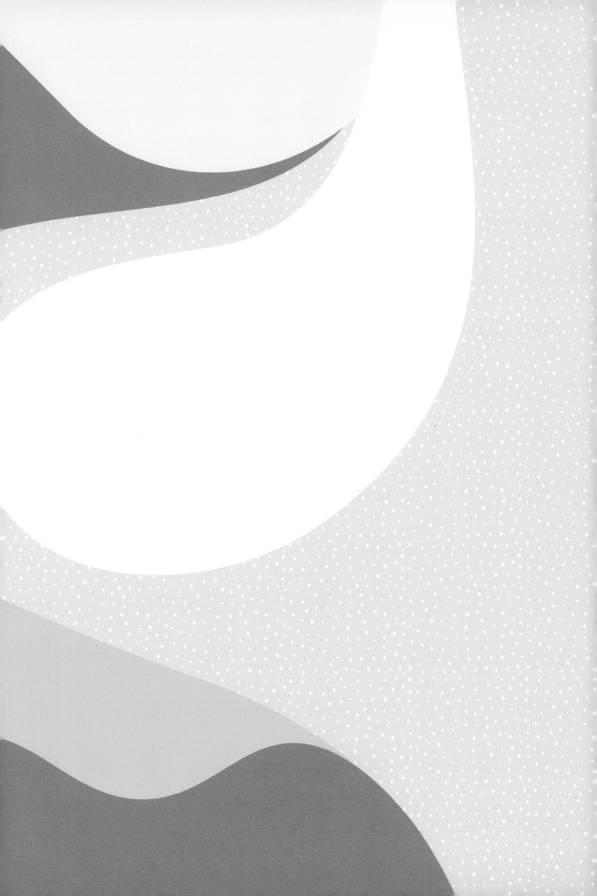

SHOES
the hunt for the perfect pair

Whether you're a heel-a-holic or a flats girl, our love affair with shoes can't be denied. And rightly so; few other accessories have the power to affect your look the way shoes can. But footwear is so much more than a question of style—due to their practical functionality, we expect our shoes to be more durable than the rest of our wardrobe. A run in your tights is a minor nuisance, whereas a broken heel can spell disaster. This is part of why vegan footwear has struggled to make its way into the mainstream: due to its "pleather" past, people hesitate to equate vegan leather with quality.

But not anymore. After in-the-know celebs such as Anne Hathaway, Olga Kurylenko, Natalie Portman, Alicia Silverstone, and Liv Tyler chose vegan shoes for the red carpet, the tide started to turn, and brands like Huntd drew women wanting to play with fashion minus the cruelty.

Repurposed materials and eco fabrics have taken over from the cheap-looking faux leather we once knew, and innovation has stepped in, offering endless possibilities. Durability is a major focus for most vegan-friendly brands. Most of them are mindful of the environment and strive to create lasting designs that won't be tossed out after just one season. Mycro, one of the most recent up-and-coming cruelty-free fabrics, is both breathable and water-resistant, crafted from a polyester substrate with a polyurethane top layer. (Note that no PVC is used in these materials, and, in many cases, they're recycled.) Birkenstock, a brand famous for its eco-friendly stance, uses two kinds of trademarked materials: Birko-Flor, made from acrylic and polyamide felt fibers, and Birkibuc, a softer version of the same.

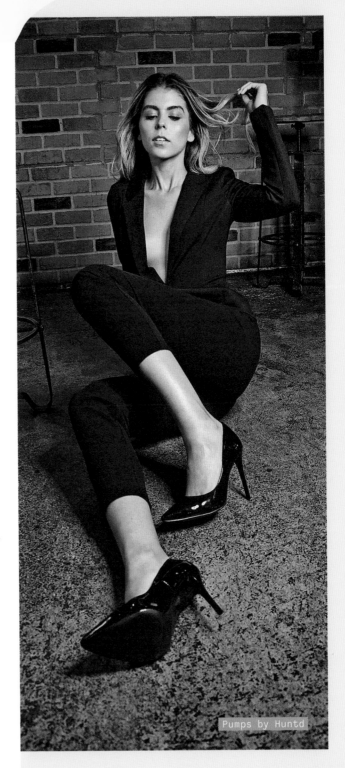

✕ ✕ ✕

Fashion's most memorable shoe moments

Naomi Campbell falling over on the runway in her Vivienne Westwood heels in 1993.

~~~

Mr. Big proposing to Carrie with a blue Manolo Blahnik shoe instead of a ring in the first *Sex and the City* movie.

~~~

Former Philippine First Lady Imelda Marcos admitting she owned more than a thousand pairs of shoes.

~~~

Daphne Guinness being the first to wear Alexander McQueen's "unwearable" Armadillo design on the red carpet.

~~~

And, of course, Dorothy clicking her red heels together in *The Wizard of Oz*.

✕ ✕ ✕

Pumps by Huntd

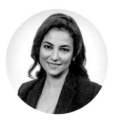

VANITA BAGRI

FOUNDER OF LABANTE LONDON

"The future is synonymous with accessible, ethical, and luxurious accessories."

The epitome of sleek and glamorous accessories, LaBante's eye-catching collections are loved by celebrities and vegan style bloggers alike. Founder Vanita Bagri hails from generations of fashion creators and, when choosing her path, opted for cruelty-free fashion. This is what she had to say:

My early experiences definitely stuck with me and shaped the brand's philosophy of fashion with respect. In my early teens, I spent many happy hours in my uncle's fashion company, watching the creation of beautiful garments for big-name brands like Calvin Klein; and therein started my love of fashion.

When I was a little older and studying at university, another pivotal moment shaped my way of thinking. I used to pass a butcher's shop where animals were kept alive and caged before being killed in front of customers for their meat. This was pretty transformative, and from that moment I became vegetarian.

After I finished my university degree, I ended up in the United States and somehow got into banking, but there was always a niggling thought that called me to combine my passion for vegetarianism with fashion. I believed there was a gap in the fashion industry for high-quality products that were not only beautiful but also cruelty-free and sustainable.

LaBante London is a labor of love, born out of a combined love of fashion, animals, and the planet. It started out really small in 2012, but grew as we received so much feedback and love from vegans, vegetarians, animal lovers, and fashionistas all over the world. As we continued to expand, we had the pleasure of meeting fashion buyers who understood that change was coming and that the future of

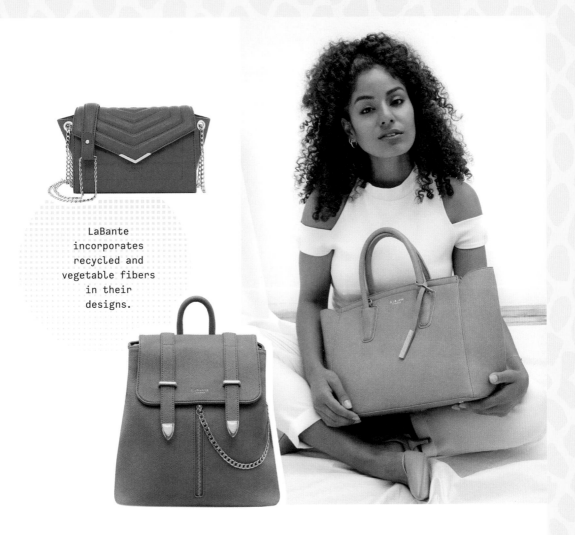

LaBante incorporates recycled and vegetable fibers in their designs.

fashion is synonymous with accessible, ethical, and luxurious accessories. Encouraged and inspired, our brand flourished, and we developed more and more beautiful and sustainable designs that were made with love to be worn with pride.

The biggest obstacle has been to find large department-store buyers and distributors for vegan fashion, as they did not initially understand how important the vegan market really was, and it has been a slow process of educating them. Slowly and surely, we began working with large chain department stores. Now, more and more of the larger ones are taking note and scheduling appointments to view our collections, and we're delighted to be working with like-minded individuals and stores who know that cruelty-free fashion is here to stay.

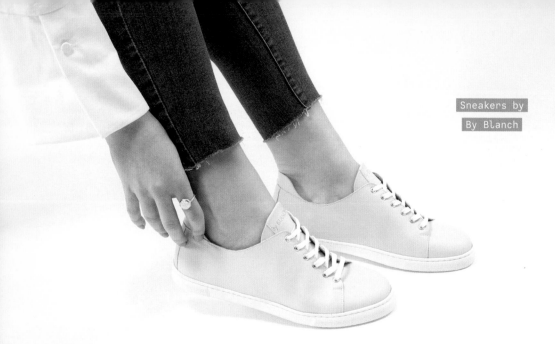

SHOES FOR ALL SEASONS
curating the ideal collection

Unlike many other fashion items, shoes are a practical matter. I'm not one of those "the higher the better" girls who chooses stilettos at any cost. When I used to see people wearing them at Milan Fashion Week—and it's always the first-timers who show up in stilettos—I noticed how they hobbled around with visibly aching feet, barely able to stand. Seasoned buyers and editors wore boots or, in more recent seasons, even sneakers. But that's not to say stilettos are to be completely eschewed. On the contrary, they will help you turn heads at that wedding, birthday party, or any event that can be traveled to via car. It's all about picking your occasions.

Much like choosing the most appropriate style for different life events, selecting the correct shoe for different weather conditions is extra challenging when you're limited in your materials. If you, like me, live in a fickle climate, you're likely to need a footwear repertoire that covers everything from fierce hail to scorching sunshine. Luckily, cruelty-free materials are always evolving, and a vast selection of vegan shoes is readily available—no matter whether you're on the lookout for winter boots or summer sandals.

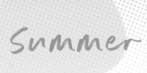
Summer

PLATFORM HEELS

Dramatic and attention-grabbing yet comfortable, platform heels are a shortcut to added height—minus the pain and discomfort. As the platform sole provides support, there is less pressure on the balls of your feet, meaning the end of that "give me flats now" feeling toward the end of the evening.
Where to find them: Nasty Gal, Susi Studio

WEDGES

Another summer classic. The wedge, much like our friend the platform, provides comfort thanks to a larger, sturdier heel that holds weight much better than its waiflike cousin, the stiletto. A colorful wedge lends a 1970s touch, while monochrome adds edge. Style yours with pretty much any summer dress or flared jeans.
Where to find them: Bourgeois Boheme

SNEAKERS

As discussed in chapter 1 (see page 16), Converse, Vans, and Supergas are a shoe gal's best friend—a welcome break from those heels, sneakers are also surprisingly easy to match. Just slip on a straight midi skirt and a simple, straightforward top and you're good to go. Sneakers are also an easy way to dress down a trench coat and sparkly accessories.
Where to find them: Zalando.com (they stock brands such as Nike and Converse and have a vegetarian shoe section), Veja, Esprit's vegan range

SANDALS
✗

When temperatures rise, the temptation to shed the boots and slip into a strappy sandal is irresistible. The ultimate wide-range shoe, sandals offer a touch of summer to any outfit, be it the smart pencil skirt or the boho maxi dress. Wear them flat for a relaxed appeal, or turn heads with skyscraper heels.
Where to find them: Esprit, Beyond Skin

Winter

KNEE-HIGH BOOTS

✗

The ultimate femme-fatale style, knee-highs may seem intimidating, but when paired with a sleek, un-bulky winter coat, they add a chic edge. Slip them on with an oversized sweater dress for cold days.
Where to find them: Lulus, Beyond Skin

CHELSEA BOOTS

✗

Versatile, comfortable, and easy to wear, Chelsea boots are the jeans of the shoe world. If you're not a huge fan of heels, or you live in an icy climate that makes platforms, knee-highs, or stilettos impractical, this will be your go-to style. Whether matched with skinny jeans or a miniskirt, they epitomize that covetable combination of sturdy and stylish.
Where to find them: Beyond Skin, Vegetarian Shoes

BIKER BOOTS

✗

From sleek to studded, biker boots have stomped their way into the wardrobes of fashionistas everywhere. Team them with a soft, unstructured coat or jacket—not faux leather, to avoid overkill.
Where to find them: Cri de Coeur

Spring/Autumn

PEEP-TOE MULES

✗

The ultimate transitional design. BHAVA Studio's founder, Francisca Pineda, has done the impossible: created the perfect trans-seasonal shoe. The sustainable footwear label has reached near-perfection with the Alden, a mule design that neatly encompasses everything I'm looking for in a shoe for the in-between seasons: it gives a wink to open-shoe weather, while not quite baring all to the degree of a sandal. It's reliable, but at the same time, sexy. It's on-trend, yet timeless. Style this design with dark skinnies and a structured jacket, or wear it with a midi dress for a city-hippie appeal.
Where to find them: BHAVA Studio

ANKLE BOOTS

✗

Possibly the most versatile shoe style out there, the ankle boot is a must-have style that will be a lifesaver through sunny spring days and rainy autumn afternoons. Style with everything from skinny jeans to minidresses.
Where to find them: By Blanch

PERFECT PUMPS
the must-own classic

There's a reason why high-heeled pumps are a must-have in any shoe wardrobe: they have the power to embody supreme sophistication and are versatile enough to range from daytime demure to after-dark seduction. After all, what other shoe lends the same polished finish to a job interview look as it does a first-date dress? Pumps are classic yet daring, the most coveted combination of them all.

A NEUTRAL HUE

As amazing as bright and neon colors are, a true everyday shoe needs to be easy to wear and match. Save the look-at-me shades for special occasions.

What to look for in your perfect pair

ROUND TOE

Pointed and square toes come and go, but a round toe will always be on-trend.

POSSIBLY A PLATFORM

For all-day comfort.

A SLIM HEEL, BUT NOT A STILETTO

The classic silhouette calls for a slim, elongated heel. However, stilettos are too dramatic and uncomfortable for frequent use.

ACCESSORIES

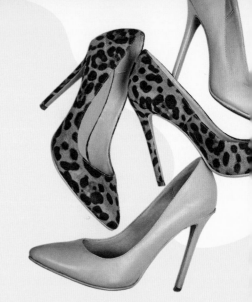

. . . AND BECAUSE SOME OCCASIONS DO CALL FOR A STILETTO

Cult of Coquette, the ultimate pair of vegan heels

At first glance, Cult of Coquette appears to be just another high-end accessory brand selling sophisticated stiletto pumps. From patent nude to leopard print, this label's versatility and elegance stands out, along with its materials. Every Cult of Coquette shoe is handmade and cruelty-free.

Inspired by timeless designs such as heel height, arch, and cut of the vamp, Cult of Coquette founder Bebe Mehr attended the Fashion Institute of Technology in New York and ran a fashion boutique for over eight years before moving to Los Angeles to found Cult of Coquette—the premium specialist in cruelty-free stilettos. She, like many others, was frustrated by the lack of vegan options when shopping for shoes. But tapping into that frustration paid off; the brand is also planning to launch a range of flats, sandals, and boots to cater to every taste and need.

Cult of Coquette's appeal lies in the design—this brand is the ultimate antidote to the tired vegan stereotype. As far from Birkenstocks as you can possibly get, Cult of Coquette is flirty, elegant, and seductive, effortlessly proving that you can succeed in staying stylish while keeping your cruelty-free values. And fashion bloggers are flocking to Cult of Coquette—the label's trademark stiletto is the ultimate statement shoe, adding flair to everything from skater dresses to ripped jeans.

Pair this head-turning design with midi skirts or skinny jeans for daytime, or team them with a sheath dress for evening—but prepare to attract attention. Wallflowers need not apply.

VEGAN STYLE

HOW TO SURVIVE
A DAY IN HEELS

Cult of Coquette founder
Bebe Mehr shares her tips

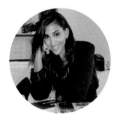

We love the extra height and "power woman" feeling that high heels can give, but let's be honest: walking in anything more than a couple of inches for too long can be a pain. Luckily, stiletto queen and Cult of Coquette founder Bebe Mehr is here to share her secrets for how to face a day in heels minus the excruciating pain and awkward wobbles:

Go for insole padding.
Cult of Coquette shoes actually have a good amount of padding. This was a conscious effort, because even many high-end designer brands have no cushioning whatsoever, and comfort is key.

~~~

Have them stretched.
Getting new shoes stretched makes a world of difference. Any shoe-repair place, and even some department stores, will offer this service. It saves your feet from having to do the dirty work, so no blisters or sore feet the first couple of times you wear new heels.

Check the toe shape.
Choosing a heel that has a toe shape that isn't too tight or constricting is also a great tip. Pointy shoes will always squeeze your toes, so you have to be aware of this before purchasing. An almond-shaped toe tends to be more comfortable, without completely sacrificing that pointy look.

~~~

Get the right extras.
Lastly, a newly discovered secret is muscle-roller balls. Rolling your feet on these balls in the mornings and evenings can really loosen your muscles and make wearing all shoes more comfortable.

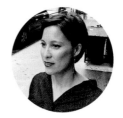

ALICIA LAI

FOUNDER OF BOURGEOIS BOHEME

"It's cool to be kind."

British brand Bourgeois Boheme was launched by designer Alicia Lai based on her ethics as a vegan. She wanted to create a brand that would be more accessible and easier for curious consumers—not just vegans or vegetarians—to find sustainable, conscious, and stylish footwear that will fit their personality and stand out from the crowd. Here, Alicia speaks about the horrors behind leather and why she was compelled to start her brand.

You don't need to be vegan to appreciate non-animal fashion, but the facts speak for themselves: the eco-friendly materials and processes available show that there's a far more innovative, desirable option than relying on animal skins. We want to educate people that ethical fashion does not only do good but is also stylish.

Beneath leather's smooth and shiny surface, there's a less attractive story.

The tanning process used to preserve animals' skin is also one of the most toxic in the world, using huge quantities of chemicals and heavy metals that pollute air, soil, and water, and can cause fatal diseases.

Animal agriculture is seriously damaging our environment. It uses 70 percent of the world's fresh water and takes up one-third of its land surface, while the intensive production of animal skins isn't just responsible for the deaths of workers involved in leather production (mostly in third-world countries) and the deaths of animals, it's polluting vast swathes of the planet and just isn't sustainable, justifiable, or necessary.

With such amazing alternative materials available, there's really no need to use animal-based products. Our shoes are lovingly crafted without any animal-derived materials such as fur, leather, wool, silk, and animal-based glues. There's absolutely no PVC either. Instead, we choose high-quality, Italian-made cotton-backed microfiber PU

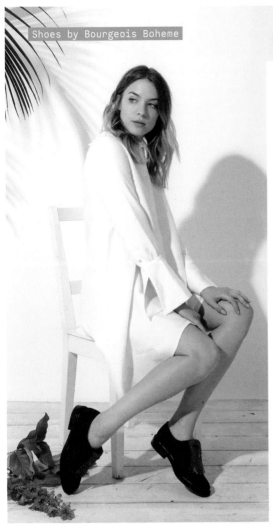

Alicia's top picks—the three styles your shoe rack cannot be without

THE CHELSEA BOOT

This versatile style keeps you warm and dry in the winter, while staying breathable and lightweight for spring.

THE SUMMER SANDAL

Ideal for city strolls as well as beach getaways.

THE BROGUE

The perfect office shoe, the brogue also lends a casual, carefree appeal to weekend outfits.

(polyurethane), textiles, and natural materials. This result is sophisticated, innovative materials that are long-lasting, super-comfortable, waterproof, and animal- and eco-friendly. What's not to love about that?

When shopping for vegan shoes, make sure the supply chain is ethical from the beginning to end of the production process and distribution. Be assured by the brand you're shopping from that the materials used for your shoes are sustainable and animal friendly. Make sure the materials are good quality so that they last a long time, and be sure to know how to take care of different materials so your shoes live happy, long lives.

HO
DESIGN A KIND ABODE

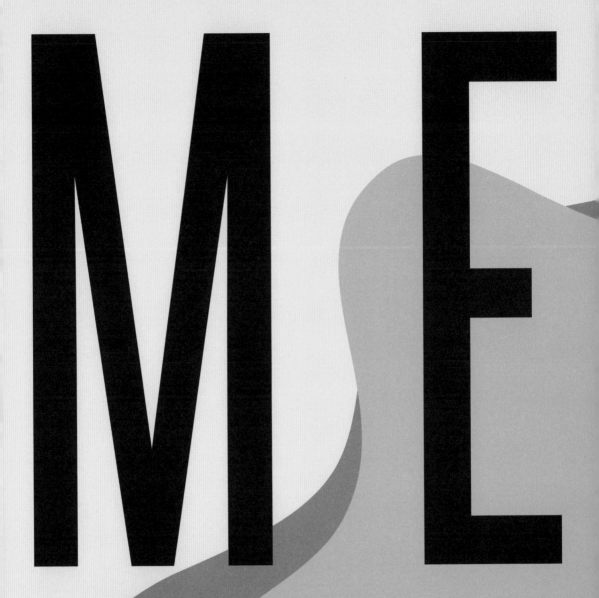

ME

Because compassionate living starts at home.

You might be an expert on plant-based diets and have started building your skin-free wardrobe,

but what about that sofa you're currently sitting on with a cup of tea, reading this? Is it made from leather? What about the pillows on your bed—are they down-filled? Chances are, your home is full of hidden animal materials.

If you've never considered homewares as part of your vegan journey, you're not alone. While food, beauty, and fashion are key areas of focus for those aiming to rid their lives of cruelly produced items, the home is often an afterthought. The vegan community is buzzing with recipes and beauty tips—and animal-friendly fashion is an up-and-coming segment—but cruelty-free living at home is still a relatively uncharted topic. Of course, if you're avoiding leather and other animal-derived materials in your wardrobe and choosing cosmetics that aren't tested on animals, it's logical that you would also want to look into making your home more cruelty-free.

The road toward creating a compassionate home can sometimes take more time than just veganizing your fridge or overhauling your beauty routine, simply because homeware items tend to pack more longevity than your average shampoo bottle—chances are slim that upon discovering your sofa is made from leather, you will immediately discard it. And you shouldn't, as randomly and carelessly throwing things away is wasteful and unnecessary. If you truly cannot bear to keep a leather chair or a wool throw in your home, give it to someone, donate it to a charity, or sell it. (I believe there's nothing wrong with selling items that you no longer use that someone else might get good use out of, but if it feels wrong to keep the money, you can always donate it to your chosen charity.) No matter how much you might want to get rid of an animal-derived furniture item in your house, keeping it is always preferable to simply throwing it out. The amount of things that we throw away contributes to large-scale waste, which is so detrimental to the planet. (Australians discard almost 500,000 tons of textiles every year. Almost 300,000 tons of textiles are thrown away in the United Kingdom every year, and the United States wastes around 15 million tons.) Remember that waste affects nature, and thus animals, on an enormous scale. Do not contribute to it if you can avoid it.

The cruelty-free transition is just that—a transition. Don't beat yourself up for not being able to afford a new sofa or simply not wanting to throw out your old one. I sat on leather sofas for years before I was gifted a faux-leather one (by my former landlady), and I didn't consider myself any less vegan because of it. Veganizing your life is a process, so let it take its time. In the meantime, get informed, read up and learn all about how to best remove animal products from your living space and what to replace them with.

COMMON ANIMAL-DERIVED FABRICS IN HOME DÉCOR
and how to replace them

You're likely to see a few recurring materials in homewares that you can easily tweak to replace with cruelty-free materials. Keep an eye out for secondhand options, which are more sustainable than newly produced faux fur and faux leather.

WOOL
v

used for

Throws, covers, and decorations.

comes from

Sheep who are often violently shorn, can sometimes be left with bleeding wounds, in some cases mulesed (see page 31), and inevitably sent to slaughter at the end of their lives. Wool is also a major contributor to global warming, as sheep are among the species that release the most methane gas into the atmosphere.

replace with

Cotton (preferably organic; see page 44), bamboo fiber, eucalyptus yarn, and linen.

FUR
v

used for

Throws and pillows.

comes from

Rabbits, foxes, mink, and many other animals that are factory-farmed in small wire cages and killed by electrocution, poisoning, or gassing, or trapped in the wild and sometimes left in agony for days before the trapper arrives and kills them, often by clubbing them to death.

replace with

Faux fur, preferably secondhand or vintage.

LEATHER AND SUEDE

used for

Furniture, such as sofas and chairs.

comes from

Mainly cows, but also sheep and sometimes dogs and cats, from China's huge dog and cat leather industry (see page 61). Over 1 billion animals per year are killed for their leather. Raising this many animals for leather is a major cause of global warming through the release of methane gas that the animals produce, and the process of turning their skins into wearable leather contributes to pollution due to the use of toxic substances. The tanning process also poisons countless workers through exposure to harsh chemicals.

replace with

Eco-friendly faux alternatives, vintage or secondhand faux leather, canvas, or fabric.

DOWN AND FEATHERS

used for

Bedding and cushions.

comes from

Ducks and geese, which are meant to be plucked only after slaughter, but plucking down from birds that are alive and conscious is very common in the industry. Despite the existence of a Responsible Down Standard, the supply chain is murky and difficult to monitor, meaning that it's pretty much impossible to be sure that you are not, in fact, relaxing under a blanket filled with feathers from live-plucked birds.

replace with

Recycled or recyclable synthetic fillers.

Giving old fibers a new life: Weaver Green

You might come across other animal materials, such as silk and angora, that are used in homewares and decorations. There is virtually no way to be sure that these products were made using animal-friendly practices, and there are many animal-free options to replace them. Look for natural materials such as cotton and linen, or recycled/recyclable synthetics. Stay on the lookout for smaller, more conscious companies that keep sustainability at the forefront of their business, such as British brand Weaver Green. This innovative label creates rugs, tote bags, cushions, and other décor materials from the recycled fibers originating from plastic pollution.

The all-vegan brand got started when founders Tasha and Barney Green were traveling through Asia and found a fishing rope made from discarded plastics. They became curious about what else could possibly be made from plastic waste, and got serious about creating a homewares collection that would help save the oceans by repurposing plastic waste. Turning plastic waste into an open fiber took time (seven years of research, to be exact) but today, Tasha and Barney are proud to offer a material that's eco-friendly as well as stain-resistant, machine washable, and can be used indoors as well as outdoors. They won a PETA award in 2018 for their wool- and down-free cushions, and their cravings-inducing online shop offers a range of eco-friendly home essentials that are handmade by artisans in Europe and Asia.

TWO INFLUENCERS
on how they created
their cruelty-free homes

When you're an influencer, showing the public your best side is literally your job—and no one knows this more than the new crop of vegan influencers, who are battling insane online competition and also choosing to profile themselves as niche tastemakers within the realm of all things vegan. And just like they create an enviable gallery of their wardrobes, meals, and travels, some influencers inspire thousands with the beauty of their home décor—which, in the cases of Dallas-based Molly Tranchin and Londoner Suszi Saunders, happens to be all vegan.

What do these stylish Instagrammers have in common? They have both won PETA awards for the impeccably chic and uniquely tasteful decoration of their living spaces. Since 2017, PETA has been giving out its Homeware Awards—a celebration of all the cruelty-free home décor options available to vegans, from big-name labels such as IKEA, Anthropologie, and Zara Home to smaller, ethically minded brands like Pacifica and Weaver Green. The variety of designs available for PETA to award is a testament to the vast availability of vegan-friendly homewares—and this is just the beginning for this compassionate industry.

But it's not only companies spearheading the change—PETA has also awarded influencers who inspired change through the eclectic and sophisticated decoration of their own homes without the use of animal materials. Read on to hear more from Molly and Suszi.

MOLLY TRANCHIN

VEGAN INFLUENCER

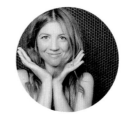

"My house is very lived-in and eclectic."

Molly Tranchin is known to her thousands of Instagram followers as vegan influencer FashionVeggie. Her account is a colorful blend of fashion, lifestyle, food, and her life as a vegan mother to a little boy. But in 2017, she became the winner of PETA's Most Stylish Cruelty-Free Home Award, showing off her gorgeous abode decorated with only vegan items. Molly's taste is authentic and eclectic, and her home in Dallas, Texas, reflects the warmth of a family feel, expertly blended with refined details. Molly explains how she veganized her home:

When I went vegan, I basically did an entire home décor overhaul. My main criteria for my new home products was that they be vegan and attractive. Pretty simple, actually, contrary to what many would think.

My house is very lived-in and eclectic. It's a huge compliment that people find it beautiful. I tend to like things with character, so I'm big on high-end thrifting. I want certain rooms to feel certain ways—for example, I want my bedroom to be soothing, spacious, and slightly cavernous. I like my living room to be cozy, glowing, and natural, with warm tones, exposed brick, wooden accents, and vegan leather. This is the room where I keep all my beloved books and knickknacks, from a driftwood and polyresin "skull" to huge geodes we picked up while on a road trip. My bathroom was made to feel spa-like, with cruelty-free and vegan products.

While I was pregnant, the most challenging item to locate was a crib mattress. So many have wool. And it did take some time to find the perfect vegan leather sofa for the living room, and to find our perfect down-alternative pillows that we love. But I wouldn't consider veganizing your

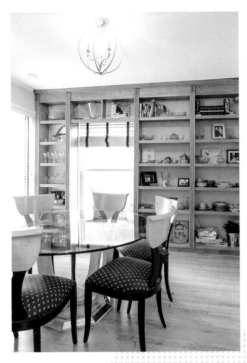

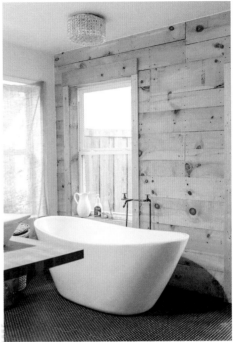

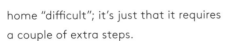

Molly's award-winning home reflects her compassionate ethics.

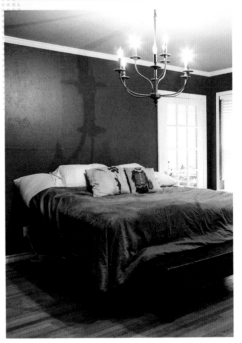

home "difficult"; it's just that it requires a couple of extra steps.

Honestly, I thrift a lot. And I love a good art gallery to add some flair to my home. But I also really like to check out Joss & Main for great deals on things like chandeliers or home accents. IKEA also has some new eco-friendly vegan pieces that I'm excited to try out.

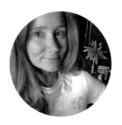

AWARD-WINNING INTERIORS
INSTAGRAMMER

"I like to mix vintage pieces with industrial, natural materials."

You'd be forgiven for thinking that Londoner Suszi Saunders is a professional interior designer—but this hypnotherapist is just a big fan of home décor, and she's incredibly good at it. When renovating her sophisticated Victorian home, Suszi decided to follow her ethics and overhauled her abode with all-vegan décor and extras. This is what she had to say:

Previously, as a big lover of texture, I had lots of sheepskin rugs strewn on floors and hanging over chairs and bannisters. I also had a lot of wool rugs and cushions with down fillings. When we moved, we took with us our two vintage leather chairs, but they were first on my list to reupholster in a vegan-friendly fabric.

Becoming vegan coincided with moving house and renovating our new home, so it gave me the perfect opportunity to start again.

I'm a huge fan of dark, inky hues. I first stumbled across this style when reading Abigail Ahern's blog. She showed how painting the ceiling, skirting boards, floors, and walls in the same dark color provided the most beautiful backdrop. I was hooked. I like to mix vintage pieces with industrial, natural materials. I also love adding a mix of metallics: silver, copper, and brass.

Adding texture is a big element in my interior design, and I found that a struggle at first. But, with a little research, I was able to find some wonderful alternatives. There are some great boho, textured cushions made from 100 percent cotton rather than wool (try Etsy, Anthropologie, Graham and Green, and Monsoon). There are also some fabulous faux-sheepskin rugs available. My favorite comes from La Redoute.

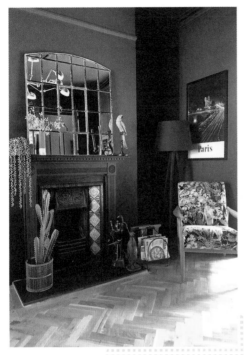

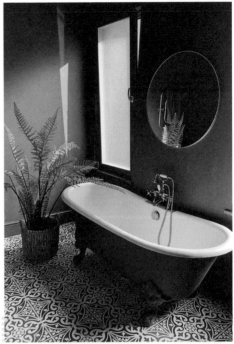

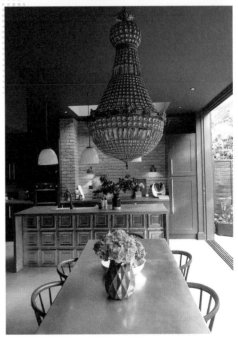

If you find something you love that isn't 100 percent vegan, reach out to the company and ask if it's possible for them to veganize it. My two velvet sofas from two different shops were, on request, stuffed with foam rather than feathers. I was also able to buy some beautiful cushion covers minus the feather fillings. The more we request cruelty-free products, the more brands will realize there's a demand.

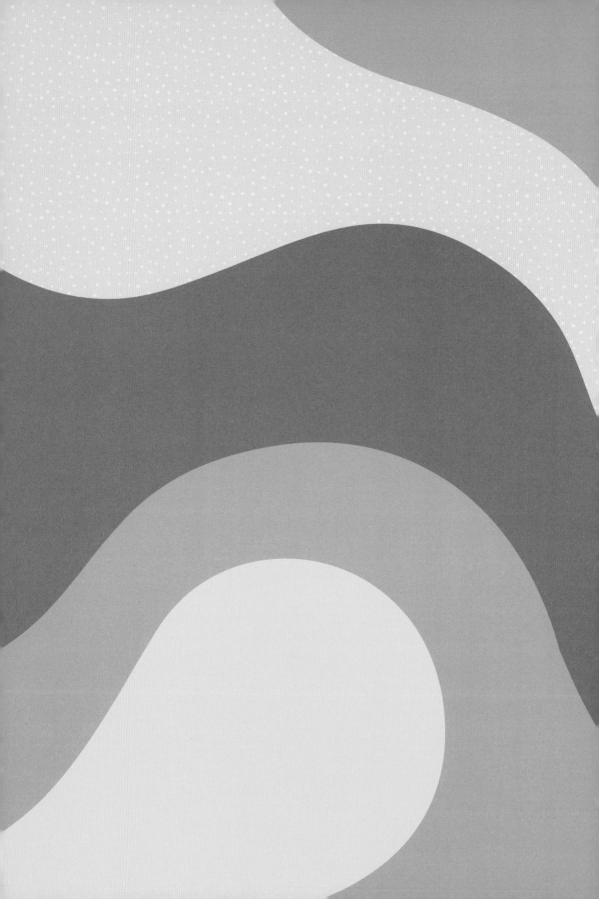

Veganizing
your life is
a process, so
let it take
its time.

A WORD ON HOME-CARE PRODUCTS

Not the most glamorous of subjects—but for most of us, cleaning our house is part of everyday life, so the products we use concern a lot of consumers. While animal testing for beauty (and medical research) has been in the public eye for years, household cleaning products are often overlooked. But if you care about keeping your cosmetics cruelty-free, then you might be interested in removing animal testing from your home, too, which means taking a better look at your home cleaning products, your fabric detergents and conditioners, and your dishwashing liquids.

As we'll discuss in chapter 4 (page 106), there is, at the time I wrote this book, a law in place in the European Union that bans cosmetics ingredients from being tested on animals in the EU (though it's not without its difficulties and loopholes). In Australia, a ban has been proposed for several years, but at the time of writing this book, it's delayed and has yet to come into effect. Cosmetics companies are currently not testing on animals in Australia, but some conduct their animal research elsewhere in the world, for the products to then be sold on the Australian market. A bill to ban animal testing for cosmetics was introduced in the United States, but has not yet passed at the time of writing this book.

Unfortunately, there is no similar ban when it comes to household products anywhere in the world, which means that it's legal to use rats, mice, guinea pigs, rabbits, and other animals in toxicity tests, carcinogenicity experiments, skin irritant tests, and many other painful experiments. In many of these tests, animals are forced to swallow or inhale large quantities of potentially toxic substances, or have harsh chemicals smeared on their skin.

Alternatives do exist. Researchers have developed methods such as 3-D tissue structures made from actual human skin to test on, along with in-vitro technologies like "organ in a chip," which uses human cells grown in a lab to mimic human organs. This is innovative, life-saving science that one day will take the place of cruel animal testing. Until then, we have to stick to good old-fashioned label reading.

Labels to look for

If you agree that cruelty to animals doesn't belong in your home, it's time to take a look at the products you're using to clean it with. Just as with beauty, there are certifications out there that allow you to know more about how your household products were made (see pages 120–21).

The eco-friendly tip: refill your bottles

The new crop of eco-friendly, zero-waste shops that are popping up in cities all over the world offer a refill service for products like household cleaners, dishwashing liquids, and fabric detergents (and sometimes shampoo, shower gel, and conditioner). So, when you've run out of your product, there's no need to throw away the bottle. Just take it to your nearest eco shop and get a refill. Most of the time, the products offered for refilling are cruelty-free and vegan (if you're not sure, always ask and check the label). This allows you to be kind to animals and the environment at the same time. Plus, you often save money—I initially worried about the price of the refills in my local ethical shop (Hisbe in Brighton, United Kingdom) but, once I went in for a refill, I realized that I had been paying more for bottled products all along. This kind of system is bound to become even more prominent in the next few years, as plastic pollution is a catastrophic problem on everyone's radar, and we increasingly strive to limit our consumption and waste.

Non-vegan ingredients lurking in your home-care products

Once you've established that the products you're using are cruelty-free, it's time to take the next step and ensure that they are vegan. (Reminder: a product is cruelty-free if it's not tested on animals. It's vegan if it doesn't have any animal-derived ingredients. See page 15.) Just like any other item you're buying, read the ingredients. Learn which ingredients aren't vegan and check the label before you buy. Here are some nasties to watch out for:

GLYCERIN

Sometimes vegan, sometimes derived from animal fat

KERATIN

A protein that comes from ground hooves, horns, feathers, and quills

LANOLIN

A substance found in sheep's wool

CARMINE

A red coloring that comes from crushed beetles (also used in beauty products)

TALLOW

A product made from animal fat

CAPRYLIC ACID

A substance derived from milk

OLEYL ALCOHOL

Comes from fish

THE DIY OPTIONS

If you're a DIY lover, you'll be pleased to find that there is a vast array of options for cleaning your home and everything in it that do not involve animal cruelty—or buying any cleaning products at all. There are items that you're likely to have in your kitchen right now that do the job just fine, such as:

VINEGAR

Just plain white vinegar, nothing fancy. Yes, the smell is a bit much, but it will get the job done, whether it's washing floors or cleaning windows. Just light a scented candle afterward (see page 105 for info on vegan-friendly ones) to get rid of the smell. Alternatively, add some essential oils or lemon to your vinegar for a more pleasant scent.

LEMON

Blend some fresh lemon juice with salt to scrub dishes and clean your kitchen, as well as wash steel utensils. A bonus point is the fresh scent.

COCONUT OIL

Not for cleaning, but a great option to add shine to your faux-leather furniture—no need for fancy leather polish. Just mix some coconut oil with the aforementioned miracle worker—vinegar—and voila, a perfect polish for your sofas and faux-leather chairs.

BICARBONATE OF SODA (BAKING SODA)

Mixed with lemon and—you guessed it—vinegar, bicarbonate of soda works wonders as a kitchen cleaner or bathroom scrub. You can even use it as a fabric conditioner in the laundry, as it helps maintain softness and boost cleanliness.

It might feel strange initially to use food products to clean your house, wash your dishes, and clean your clothes, but after you've been doing it for a while, it will start feeling exactly what it is—natural. If you're ever faced with using industrial cleaners again, you'll probably find yourself flinching at their chemical smells and unnatural feel.

CHLOE BULLOCK

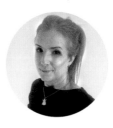

VEGAN INTERIOR DESIGNER,
MATERIALISE INTERIORS

"I have always encouraged clients to make ethical choices."

Interior designer Chloe Bullock is based in Brighton, United Kingdom, and worked as a designer for The Body Shop for a decade before starting her own compassionate design business, Materialise Interiors, where she works with vegan and non-vegan clients alike on creating beautiful spaces without the use of animal skins. Chloe has worked with restaurants, shops, and commercial spaces on creating a signature look for their space, always trying to influence her clients to choose vegan-friendly materials. Chloe explains how her background in design influenced her business:

I studied Furniture and Product Design at Nottingham Trent University. Upon graduating, one of my final projects won Consumer Product Design of the Year at New Designers—a show that, each year, brings together the best from the design courses across the United Kingdom. Subsequently, I worked as a designer for a local furniture company before spending ten years specifying and designing ethically sourced interiors for The Body Shop International globally.

I have actually had my interior design business, Materialise Interiors, for over twelve years, but only certified it as a vegan business recently, with a certification from VeganDesign.org, which also included a course to specialize as a vegan design business. The prompt was listening to LuAnn Nigara's *A Well-Designed Business* podcast when she was interviewing VeganDesign.org founder Deborah DiMare. I really thought I had a handle on the industry from my Body Shop days—it struck me that there was an awful lot that I wasn't aware of. Wool and down were the biggest shocks to me.

I've been designing vegan interiors for years without formally pointing it out to clients. I will work for any client if the project and fit is right, rather than saying I only work on vegan projects—I feel it's better to have discussions on specifications as they come up and show clients how vegan alternatives are better. Increasingly, these vegan alternatives are better-performing and cheaper, so it's getting easier to convince clients.

I have always encouraged clients to make ethical choices when specifying their projects. I want to spread the word, so I've promoted my vegan design speciality to raise awareness and hopefully get other designers to take the course and educate themselves.

CHLOE'S ADVICE FOR VEGANIZING YOUR HOME

Animal products harbor far more dust and mites, which is unhealthy, especially for allergy sufferers, so vegan products can even help to improve your health.

~~~

The wool industry is cruel, and the use of wool in interiors is being superseded by better-performing synthetic materials, minus the animal abuse.

~~~

Leather does not perform well. If it's from China, it may not just be bovine (see page 61), and tannery workers spend their days inhaling toxic chemicals, which can lead to fatal diseases.

Feathers and down are not traceable, and there is no such thing as "ethical" feathers, as the chain of custody is not reliable. I hadn't realized that down and angora were live-harvested. It's gruesome, and often the animals die from the pain.

Chloe's top vegan-friendly alternatives:

Sunbury Design does contract-quality leather, suede, and wool alternatives, which I've been using for more than a decade. They're my favorite.

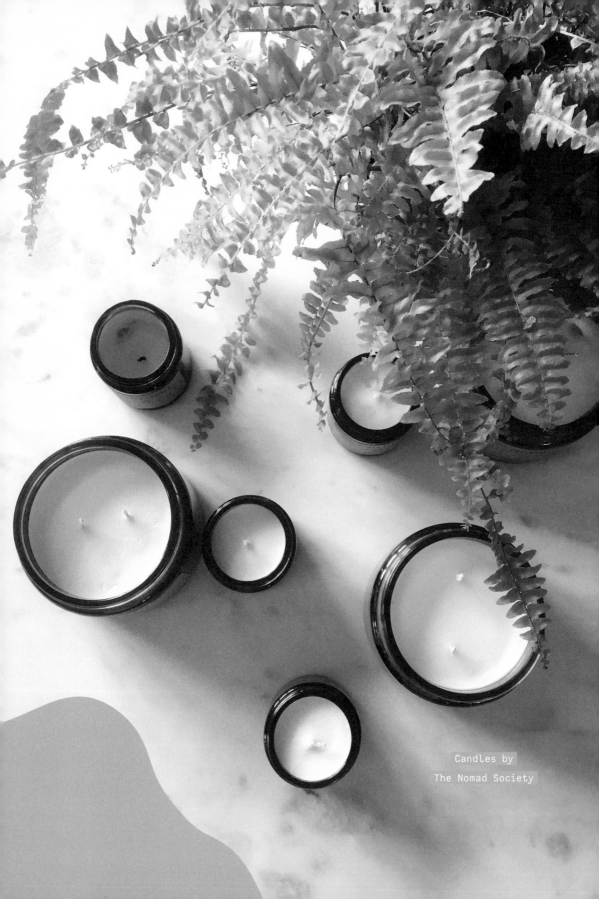

Candles by
The Nomad Society

MAKING SCENTS
of home fragrance

Nothing sets an atmosphere and creates warmth within a home like the comforting fragrance of a scented candle. If you, like me, are a serial hoarder of scented candles (raise your hand if you're a fellow lover of cinnamon and vanilla), you might already know that there are two main options for conventionally made candles: beeswax and paraffin. One is non-vegan, the other is technically vegan but problematic for a variety of reasons. Another seemingly vegan product is palm wax, which comes with its own set of issues.

Beeswax is produced by bees (duh) and is a honey by-product. It's made by melting a honeycomb with the use of boiling water. The animal-rights issues with beeswax are the same ones that we face when it comes to honey. Farmers at honey farms often forcibly impregnate bees and sometimes remove the queen bee's wings to keep her from leaving the colony. Bees make honey for themselves to survive the winter, but farmers substitute it with cheap sugar water that lacks the nutrition that honey offers the bees. Bees are necessary to our ecosystem, and despite the fact that they're small, they're sentient animals just like cows, pigs, or dogs, so compassionate humans should do their best to protect them. Thankfully, beeswax, which is also quite expensive, is not necessary at all to produce candles.

Paraffin is the cheaper option and the ingredient that makes up the majority of commercially produced candles, especially those on the cheaper end of the spectrum. It's a petroleum by-product, which, on its own, makes it a problematic choice for those who want to make their home as eco-friendly as possible. Studies have also shown that paraffin candles release chemicals such as the known carcinogens benzene and toluene into the environment where they burn. Yikes. If you want to create an inviting atmosphere in your home without the toxic air pollution, then paraffin might not be the ideal choice.

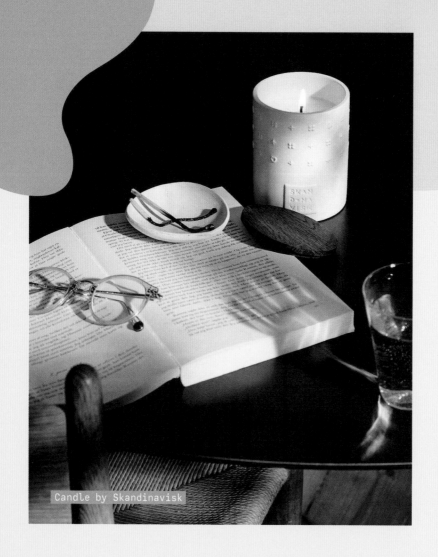

Candle by Skandinavisk

Palm wax is derived from palm oil, which you will, without a doubt, have heard of. When it was first used for candles, it was actually seen as the "sustainable" alternative to paraffin. It's a cheap ingredient that you will generally find hard to avoid, as it's present in so many food products. But, as the much-discussed palm oil debate has shown, palm oil production is responsible for deforestation on a massive scale, which obviously includes habitat destruction and the displacement of animals from their homes. So, while palm oil might technically be a plant-derived product, the ethics around its use are certainly questionable.

VEGAN STYLE

The vegan and ethical alternatives

SOY WAX

●

Ah, the versatile soybean. We enjoy it as milk in our tea, we stuff our faces with sausages made from it, and now we can also make candles from it. Soy is a true vegan superhero! Candles made from soy wax are eco-friendlier, as soya is a renewable resource, and it's also naturally biodegradable. If you're avoiding GMO soy in your food, you might want to look for GMO-free soy candles as well.

Where to find it: Harper's Candles, Pacifica, Sensory Soy, Vegan Bunny, Little Soap Company, Bliss Candles

COCONUT WAX

●

This newbie on the block is made from another vegan superhero product: the coconut, used for everything from coconut milk in your coffee to coconut oil that doubles as lip balm. Coconut wax is free from the cruelty of beeswax, the deforestation issues of palm oil, and the GMO concerns of soy. It's made by blending coconut oil with other waxes, often vegetable (see below), and the coconut smell is removed prior to this process so that all coconut-wax candles do not actually smell of coconut. It provides a clean and slow burn, often with a longer burn time than other waxes. However, the downside is that it may be more expensive than soy, palm, paraffin, or vegetable waxes.

Where to find it: Cocomoon, Epiphany Candles, Aloha Bay, Cocolux Australia, Evermore London

VEGETABLE WAX

●

This generic name encompasses several types of waxes, including palm and coconut, that all come from plants. Vegetable-blend waxes are often made from different oils, such as rapeseed oil, and sometimes blended with soy in a hydrogenating process that basically solidifies oil into wax. These are a more natural option than paraffin, and arguably more sustainable, as they come from renewable sources. Plus, you don't have to worry about toxicity and air pollution like you do with paraffin candles. If palm oil or GMO soy are a concern, read the label and avoid.

Where to find it: The Nomad Society, Skandinavisk, Osmology, Bare Naturals

BEA

LOOK GOOD, DO GOOD

UTY

Everything you
need to know about
looking gorgeous
while staying
cruelty-free.

When you make the switch to cruelty-free living,

your relationship with your makeup and beauty products will rapidly switch from "just slap it on in the morning" to a deeper, more inquisitive "What's in it?," "Where does it come from?," and, perhaps most important, "How was it tested?" You will probably stop shopping for beauty products at the drugstore or the supermarket and start browsing online, at health stores, and in specialty shops. That's not to say that all mainstream sources of beauty products are off-limits: British chain Superdrug has an amazing own-brand range of cruelty-free and vegan beauty products, for example. But let's just say you may need to broaden your horizons.

You will, without a doubt, discover a myriad of new brands and products that you had no idea about, and, most likely, you'll be amazed at how much choice there is and how many amazing brands are out there that no one knows or talks about. I know that when I first went cruelty-free, I wanted to shout from the rooftops about some of the stuff I found. "How come no one knows about these brands?" I would think while flipping through my favorite glossy magazines. "Why is none of this stuff in here?" Today I still skim through the beauty pages in magazines, but they mainly tend to focus on big-name brands that engage in animal testing. These days, we have the Internet to share information, and digital word-of-mouth is a powerful tool. All of a sudden, niche beauty brands are growing thanks to the enthusiastic words of consumers—and many of them are vegans, a very outspoken crowd on the Internet.

There are two things you should consider while shopping for beauty products as a vegan: Has the product been tested on animals? And does it contain any animal ingredients?

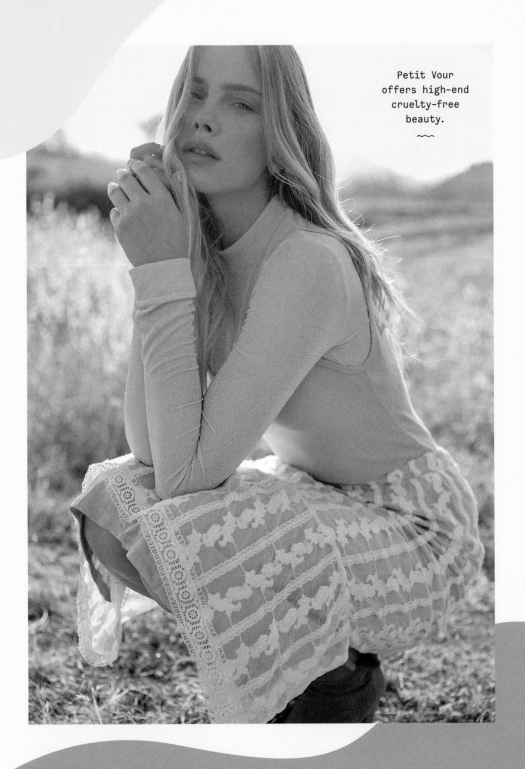

Petit Vour
offers high-end
cruelty-free
beauty.
~~~

BEAUTY

What does "cruelty-free" REALLY MEAN?

The term "cruelty-free" is meant to mark a product that hasn't been or doesn't contain ingredients that have been tested on animals. Unfortunately, animal testing is still widely used in the world, and in some countries like China, it's mandatory by law. In 2013, a ban came into place in Europe, meaning that no cosmetics or ingredients could be tested on animals. This landmark ban was an incredible statement by the European Union, making it clear that testing on animals and making money from it is unacceptable. India and Israel followed soon after with bans of their own. In Australia, a ban has been proposed for several years—prompting celebration from animal rights activists— but at the time of writing this book, the ban is delayed and has yet to come into effect. Cosmetics companies are currently not testing on animals in Australia, but some conduct their animal research elsewhere in the world, for the products to then be sold on the Australian market. A bill to ban animal testing for cosmetics was introduced in the US, but has not yet passed at the time of writing.

But—and this is an important "but"—there are quite a few loopholes in the incredibly complicated EU law. Contrary to what you might immediately conclude, the ban does not mean that it is now okay to gallop off to the beauty counter and go straight for the mainstream brand you know and love. The ban forbids companies from testing products and ingredients in the EU and from selling animal-tested products and ingredients in the EU. It also forbids companies from testing products and ingredients on animals *elsewhere* and selling them in the EU. What it doesn't keep companies from doing is testing products and ingredients on animals outside the EU and selling them outside the EU. This makes it completely possible for companies to profit from testing on animals, as long as they don't do it within the EU.

And this is where certain non-EU markets come into play—namely, China: a gigantic market—possibly the biggest in the world—where testing on animals is compulsory by law. In order to be considered truly cruelty-free, a brand must ensure that none of their products or ingredients are tested on animals. And this can only be done one way: by refusing to sell in China.

Obviously, not every beauty brand under the sun will be ready and willing to give up a market of that size. China is a lucrative chunk of the globe, and most brands will pretend to solve this sticky issue by putting a disclaimer somewhere on their website that says that they "do not test on animals unless required by law." The unwitting customer is likely to think, "Hey, it's the law—the companies are doing their best." What the companies conveniently omit is that they could, in theory, simply avoid selling in markets where such testing is required by law and thus stay cruelty-free at all times—which, of course, they aren't happy to do, as that would cost them.

The solution to this dilemma? Always do your research (you've learned this by now, haven't you?) and check whether the company whose lipsticks and moisturizers you're lusting after sells their stuff in China. If the answer is yes, then I hate to break it to you, but as of right now, in 2019, there is no way this brand and its products are cruelty-free no matter how much they claim they are on their website. (Look out for the "except when required by law" disclaimer—that's your clue.) Because they have a choice, and that is not to sell in China.

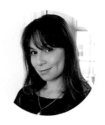

EDEN DI BIANCO

VEGAN MAKEUP ARTIST

"It makes me excited and hopeful that we can help successfully lobby major brands to push for animal-testing reforms."

Licensed cosmetologist Eden Di Bianco counts co-creator of *The Daily Show* Lizz Winstead and JCPenney among her clients, as well as vegan fashion brands VAUTE and Brave GentleMan. She told me how it all started:

I can remember having an interest in hair and makeup from a very young age. I was fascinated with my mother's frosted eyeshadows in the 1980s, gleefully destroyed my own brows in the late 1990s, and found my perfect shade of signature red in the early 2000s.

When Kevyn Aucoin's books hit the scene in the late nineties, it was life-changing for me and so many others I know. My older sister got me *Making Faces* for my birthday, and that book, along with the influences of the *Club Kids* and artists I knew, really prompted me to pursue cosmetology for a living.

I started out in a corporate, nine-to-five environment, but always in the back of my mind was my love of beauty. When the market crashed (in 2008), I was painfully unhappy in my role and decided it was time to pursue my passion and attend cosmetology school. There, I met artist Timoria McQueen, who was also in the program. She encouraged me to pursue makeup alongside hair and gave me advice and opportunities to assist her.

The very first foundations I bought to practice with were from the drugstore. I was filling in for a friend doing makeup at a strip club, which was sometimes hilarious and great practice in building my application speed and in creating looks that really hold up to sweat and long wear—it might be how and why I now specialize in bridal and special-event looks. Soon after, I got my hands on foundations from OCC (Obsessive Compulsive Cosmetics) and started to build my cruelty-free kit.

It took me a very long time and constant tweaking, but I now have a full kit that I love. I have a definite highlighter problem and every type of foundation medium known to man: liquid, powder, cream, silicone-based, water-based, alcohol-based, wax-based, airbrush, hand-applied—all entirely vegan.

For most people, the switch to cruelty-free comes after they've watched a documentary or seen a social media post about the cruelty of animal vivisection for cosmetics. Instead, for me, it was my starting point.

Animal welfare, rescue, and advocacy have been important elements of my life from a young age. I have a rescue pit bull named Frankie Beans. He's an old guy now, nearly thirteen. We've had him most of his life, and he's my whole heart. We also had lots of pets growing up, and having a deep relationship with my companion animals laid the foundation for my cruelty-free beauty practice. Animal vivisection for cosmetic products is so incredibly cruel and unnecessary. We've made such advances in research and developed testing methods that are safer, more accurate, and more humane, and it's a crime against decency that these methods are not universally used.

I've had mixed reactions from other artists in the cosmetology community. However, more and more, I meet people who are seeking cruelty-free options or are switching to exclusively cruelty-free products. It makes me excited and hopeful that, as an industry, we can help successfully lobby major brands and conglomerates to use their financial resources to push for animal testing reforms and humane regulations in markets like China.

The term "cruelty-free" isn't uniformly applied in cosmetology, and can cause confusion among consumers and makeup artists alike. Many feel that by supporting cruelty-free brands— whether or not their parent companies also endorse cruelty-free—they are demonstrating enough of a demand for these products to increase the market share. Others take it a step further and consider something "cruelty-free" only if the brand, parent company, and any third-party contributors are also cruelty-free and vegan.

Personally, I don't use brands that identify as cruelty-free but whose parent companies allow animal testing. To me, this discredits the commitment of the brand. As a result, I've had to reduce the range of products that I use and take time to find replacements. Of all my products, though, the one that's easiest to find in high-quality, cruelty-free options is foundation. Every foundation I stock is cruelty-free, and the overwhelming majority are also vegan.

Cruelty-free
beauty dictionary:
the ingredients
that you didn't
know came
from animals

While most of us know
the meaning of words such
as beeswax, you could be
forgiven for not knowing
what ambergris or carmine
is. Here are a few more
ingredients that you
might want to be aware
of next time you're at
the beauty counter.

AMBERGRIS

comes from the oil that lines whales'
stomachs (yes, really) and is often
present in perfumes.

BEESWAX

is obviously produced by bees and is
a coproduct of the honey industry.
Can be found in face creams, lip balms,
lotions, and mascara.

CARMINE

comes from crushing little red insects
called *Dactylopius coccus*. Often used
as a colorant in lipsticks.

ESTROGEN

are female hormones taken from the urine
of pregnant female mammals. Used as an
ingredient in perfumes and lotions.

VEGAN STYLE

FISH SCALES are often used to lend a shimmery effect to eyeshadows and highlighters. Next time you want to add some sparkle, just make sure your products are vegan.

GUANINE is a shimmering, light-diffusing material found in crushed fish scales. Used in mascara, lipstick, and nail polish.

KERATIN is something you will see as an active ingredient in many hair treatments. It's actually the ground hooves, horns, and hair of a variety of mammals.

LANOLIN is a sweaty, fatty excretion (nice, huh?) found on wool-bearing animals that's used in makeup remover and moisturizers.

MUSK OIL is mistakenly referred to as a plant oil, but it's actually a secretion from musk deer, musk rat, beaver, or otter genitals. Not what you want in your perfume.

SQUALENE comes from shark livers and is present in lipstick and eye makeup.

TALLOW is animal fat, which comes from boiled animal carcasses. Foundations, eyeshadows, and lipsticks often contain tallow.

BEAUTY

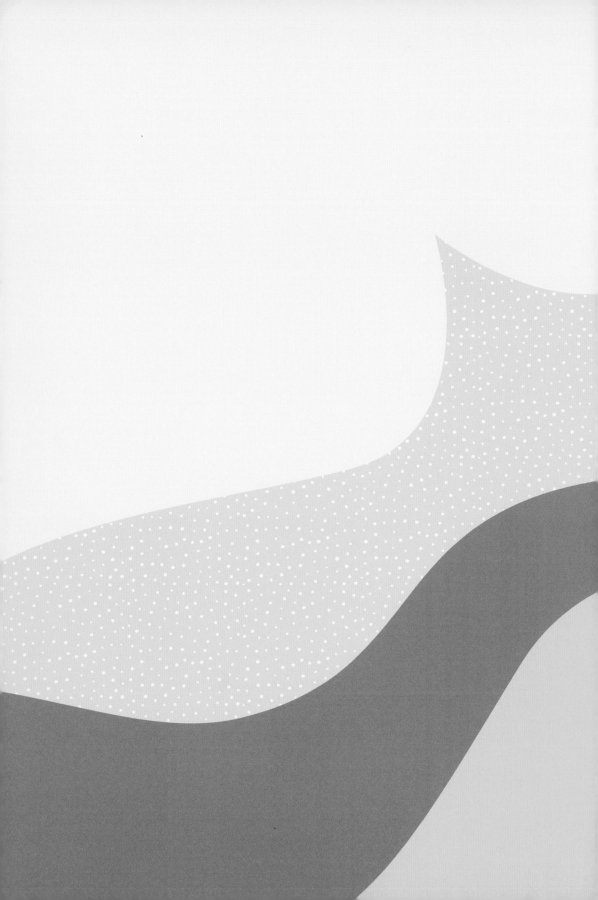

There are two things you should consider when shopping for beauty products as a vegan: Has the product been tested on animals? And does it contain any animal ingredients?

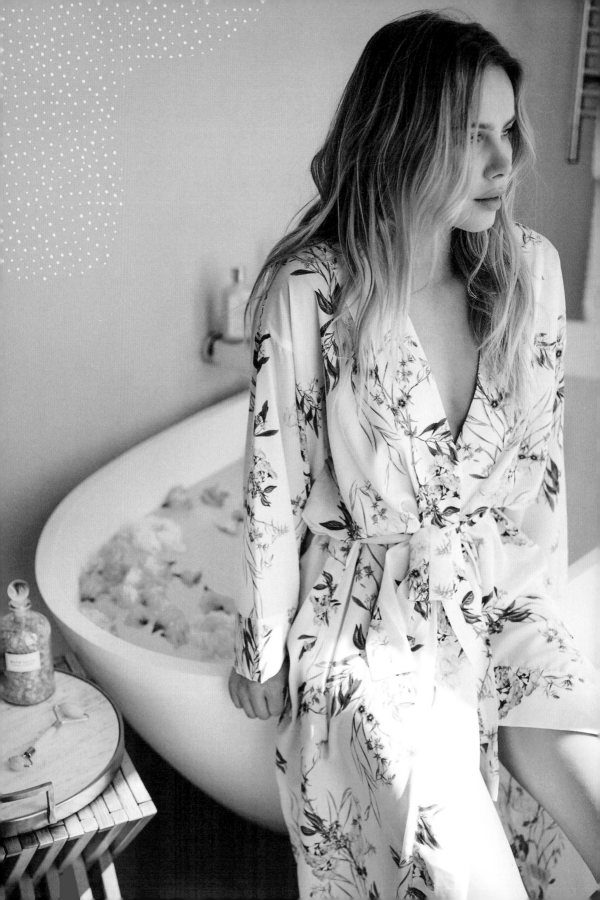

Your animal-friendly BEAUTY CABINET

So, now that you know the rules and what to avoid, how do you overhaul your beauty collection? My advice is to make the switch gradually. There's something daunting about tossing out your entire assortment of beauty products at once, but you can pledge to start shopping cruelty-free from now on. Research every new product you buy. Check the ingredients and read up on what those words actually mean.

THE LOGOS TO TRUST

We've already discussed the fact that it's anything but easy to know who and what to trust when it comes to identifying what is cruelty-free and what isn't. That's why I wanted to go through a few symbols that you can look out for on packaging.

First of all, a disclaimer: a company doesn't need any logos to be cruelty-free. It's perfectly possible for a company to sell cruelty-free products without sporting any logos on their packaging. For example, LUSH is a company that's known for their cruelty-free stance. Their vegan products (which make up the majority of their range) are certified by The Vegan Society, but they carry no official cruelty-free logo, as they have their own certification process to ensure that none of their products or ingredients are tested on animals.

For many brands, the issue with featuring a logo is that there are not only fees to pay to sign up to the charities' cruelty-free programs but also a long verification process in order to qualify. There are also extra fees to be able to feature the logo on the packaging. So, even if a brand is certified by an association, you may not always see the logo when you buy their products. Always check the databases provided by the association or organization that issued the logo.

LEAPING BUNNY BY CRUELTY FREE INTERNATIONAL

Cruelty Free International is the best known and largest international organization for the abolition of testing on animals. They work against the testing of ingredients in cosmetics and household products, and also against medical research on animals. To make things easier for compassionate shoppers, they have created the Leaping Bunny certification—a logo that exists to assure the customer that the cosmetic or household product they are buying is, in fact, cruelty-free.

To find out if a brand or product qualifies for the Leaping Bunny logo, Cruelty Free International audits its entire supply chain, from ingredient provenance to the finished product. To become Leaping Bunny certified, companies must:

O Guarantee that neither their finished products nor any ingredients used in these products have been tested on animals at any point in their development after a fixed cut-off date;

O Actively oversee their supply chains, receiving yearly guarantees that no animal testing has been done after the cut-off date;

O Agree to an audit of their supplier monitoring system by an independent organization.

To help customers find Leaping Bunny–certified products, Cruelty Free International has an easy-to-use list on their website where you can search for cosmetics or household products to find brands that don't test on animals.

BEAUTY WITHOUT BUNNIES BY PETA

The world's largest animal rights group, PETA, needs no introduction. Having made miles and miles of progress in promoting a vegan diet and animal-free fashion, PETA is also a pioneer when it comes to helping compassionate shoppers choose products that aren't the result of cruelty. How? One of their tools is their Beauty Without Bunnies program. If you are US-based, this is the most trustworthy logo.

PETA not only list companies that do *not* test on animals; they also list the ones that *do*, just to take the guesswork out of it. On their website, you can search by country and also see the countries working for regulatory change—i.e., working to change the industry from within and send the message that cruelty-free beauty is worth investing in.

CHOOSE THE CRUELTY FREE RABBIT

Australian-based organization Choose Cruelty-Free (CCF) has created this symbol in Australia to accredit cosmetics, toiletries, and household-product companies that wish to certify their ranges as cruelty-free. CCF's work includes:

o Advocating that companies use a cruelty-free ethic;

o Reviewing and accrediting companies using some of the strictest criteria in the world;

o Producing the CCF list of accredited brands and products to make shopping easier for consumers;

o Producing the CCF logo (the rabbit above), which companies can use in their branding materials.

Below are some of the criteria CCF uses for its accrediting purposes. The company cannot use an ingredient that:

o Comes from an animal killed for that purpose;

o Was forcibly and painfully extracted from an animal;

o Comes from wildlife;

o Is a by-product of the fur industry;

o Is a commercially viable product that comes from the slaughterhouse industry (even if an animal was not killed specifically to obtain it).

CCF will not accredit companies unless the parent company *and* the subsidiary are accredited. To be accredited, a company must follow these rules for all ingredients:

o The never-tested rule: None of its products or product ingredients have been tested on animals by it, its suppliers, or anyone on their behalf;

o The five-year (or more) rolling rule: None of its products or product ingredients have been tested on animals by it, its suppliers, or anyone working on their behalf within the five years immediately preceding the date of application for accreditation.

BEAUTY

HAIR

LUSH I Love Juicy

The perfect glossy-mane remedy. You don't need any fancy serums or other expensive products when you've got the supreme, get-it-clean super-tool that is I Love Juicy.

BODY CARE

Grown Alchemist Intensive Body Cream

This Australian minimalist vegan label is known for its organic range. This super-hydrating cream is made with rosa damascena, acai, and pomegranate.

THE BEAUTY MUST-HAVES

Now that you know the basics of cruelty-free shopping, here are the best vegan-friendly beauty and self-care products that will revolutionize your beauty cabinet.

SKINCARE

The Body Shop Aloe Soothing Day Cream

Aside from being ridiculously affordable, this skin-saver contains aloe vera, which will keep breakouts at bay and help your skin stay clear, smooth, and hydrated.

LIPS

Beauty Without Cruelty Natural Infusion Lipstick

It glides on, moisturizes your lips, and lasts a solid few months. And it's completely free from animal-derived ingredients. My signature color is no. 52, Cerise.

MASCARA

Urban Decay Perversion Mascara

Promising "bigger, blacker, badder" lashes, this vegan mascara actually delivers.

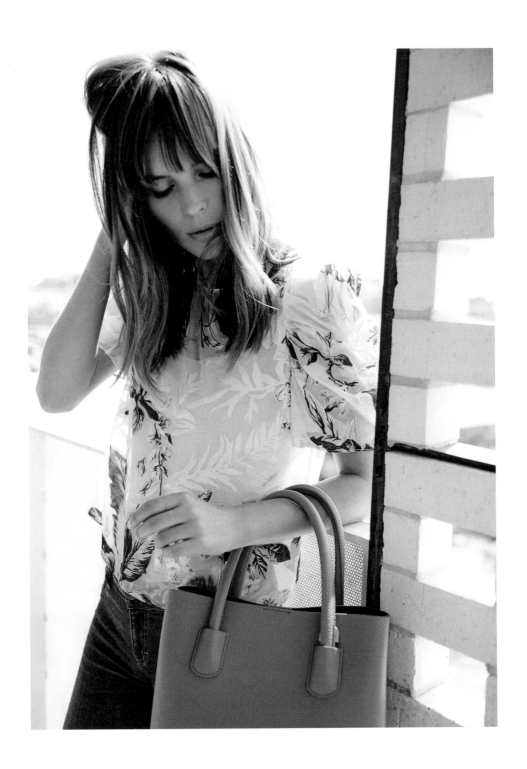

123

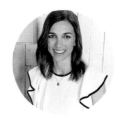

MADELINE ALCOTT

FOUNDER OF PETIT VOUR VEGAN BEAUTY BOX

"My mission is to share products that are so amazing that vegans and non-vegans flock to stock up."

When beauty subscription boxes hit the market, many vegans and cruelty-free consumers were disappointed as there was no way to know whether the products offered were tested on animals or not. Luckily, entrepreneur Madeline Alcott came to the rescue by offering a chic, luxurious, and indulgent monthly subscription box featuring only compassionate products. Petit Vour brings you the "crème de la cruelty-free" every month. Madeline explains more about her background here:

The years following my graduation from the University of Texas at Austin, I worked and traveled, moving from city to city, seeking life inspiration from new environments—Jakarta, Portland, Baltimore, Houston, and San Francisco, to name a few. Living out of a suitcase

and pushing myself to the limit cemented my belief that happiness comes from challenging, mission-driven work. I hadn't found the perfect mission-driven fit, so I set out to create something purposeful of my own.

As a self-proclaimed ingredient-sleuth, I already had years of product and industry research under my belt. It was just a matter of taking my research and developing it into something useful and innovative for conscious consumers. Petit Vour began to manifest shortly after the idea came to me, and I sprang into action. Being the first vegan beauty box, our subscription base grew quickly into a few thousand subscribers, and, after our first year in business, my partner joined in on the evolving venture: me running the front-end business and social media, him running the back-end web design and coding.

Petit Vour is a two-part business that seamlessly blends the monthly box and the shop. The monthly box is a subscription service that lets you sample the crème de la cruelty-free, curated to your beauty profile. The box is all about discovery—a celebration of natural beauty, consciously crafted and created to deliver results. The cherry-picked samples allow subscribers to get a feel for our most trusted brands, without having to commit to full-size.

There are thousands of beauty brands out there, and more are launching every day, so sifting through them to find the best is the most challenging process we face day-to-day. Brands needs to use clean, vegan ingredients and ethical manufacturing with zero animal testing. We're also looking for new and exciting products that have beautiful branding.

Since there's an ongoing need to fill each month's box with new brands and products, it can be tempting for any beauty box company to relax their standards to make sure they can get enough products and cheap deals. Since our mission is to help people discover the best of vegan beauty, having unbreakable standards is essential, and it has helped us form a strong trust with our customers and brands.

Before connecting with a brand, I go through my mental checklist. They must be cruelty-free and not be associated with any parent company that tests on animals or sells in China, where animal testing is required by law. They must also offer vegan options and have a clear mission to provide cleaner cosmetics. We don't just want products that are 100 percent vegan—we want products that are vegan *and* made with healthy ingredients that most certainly don't cause any harm to our bodies. From that point, I focus on aesthetics and performance. The brand has to be lovely enough to be displayed on the vanity or else it won't be well-received by our audience. Then, of course, products must do as they promise. A vegan product that doesn't do the job doesn't help the vegan beauty movement at all. My mission is to share products that are so amazing that vegans and non-vegans flock to stock up.

We feature only brands that are at the forefront of luxury green beauty: Kypris, Lily Lolo, Juice Beauty, Meow Meow Tweet, 100% Pure, One Love Organics, Suntegrity, Josh Rosebrook— I could go on! Petit Vour is made for savvy green beauty lovers, and it's important that we keep our standards very high.

THE SCENT OF CRUELTY-FREE
meet organic perfumery Eden

We've all been there: you're standing in the duty-free shop at the airport, having a whiff of some lovely fragrances . . . and then walking away because, as they are neither vegan nor cruelty-free, you can't entertain the idea of buying one. But what if you could have the designer perfumes you love without the nasty chemicals and the cruelty? That's exactly what Eden Perfumes, a Brighton-based family business, is achieving. Born from the idea of entrepreneur Jacqueline Moya and her partner, as well as her vegan Spanish–Mexican family, Eden Perfumes offers an endless range of fragrances that take you as far from hemp and patchouli as humanly possible. We're talking luxurious, indulgent scents—the ones you're used to finding in glossy perfume shops. Only these fragrances are free from any nasty chemicals or animal-based ingredients.

The idea behind this organic perfume house is to take the designer scents that you know and love from your pre-vegan days and replicate them with no toxic ingredients—we're talking no parabens, no phthalates, no animal-derived ingredients, and no animal testing—by blending essential oils into handmade, artisanal perfume blends. That's right—no need to give up that Chanel No. 5 scent just because you're now living the cruelty-free life. I should know—I'm frequently a fan of the no. 9, inspired by Ralph Lauren Blue, for summer, and the no. 62, reminiscent of Armani Si, for winter.

Eden perfumes come in male, female, and unisex versions, and if you ever end up in one of their three shops in the south of England, it will take you ages to sniff through all the amazing scents on offer to find The One. But once you do, you'll love it—mine lasts all day, and once you run out, you can go back to the shop for a refill, so the glass bottle isn't wasted.

Another plus is that Eden perfumes are surprisingly affordable for their high quality—a middle-sized bottle that lasts around six months is very affordable.

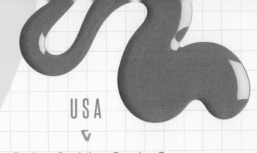

WHERE TO GET GLOSSY
the directory

Whether you're a world traveler or just on the hunt for new cruelty-free places in your area, here are a few fabulous, ethical salons around the globe where you know your treatments will be free from animal ingredients and testing.

SWEDEN

Ecohair, Södra Agnegatan 28, Stockholm (ecohair.se)

GERMANY

Hair Studio Weinhönig, Kopenhagener Strasse 75, 2nd floor, Berlin (weinhönig.de)

UK

The Rabbit Hole Organic Vegan Hair Parlour, 6A Charleville Road, London (therabbitholelondon.com)
Cuttlefish Salon, 31 Gloucester Road, Brighton (cuttlefishecosalons.com)
The Styling Lounge, 15–29 Union Street, Bristol (thestylinglounge.co.uk)

USA

The Parlour St. Johns Cruelty-Free Hair, 7327 N Charleston Avenue, Portland, Oregon (theparlourstjohns.com)
Crop Salon, 521 N Avenue 64, Los Angeles, CA (cropsalon.com)
The Green Spa & Wellness Center, 8804 Third Avenue, Brooklyn, New York (greenspany.com)

AUSTRALIA

Naturally Organic Hair Salons (PETA-certified): Brisbane, Carindale, Indooroopilly and Chermside (organichairsalons.com.au)
That Vegan Hairdresser, 129 Princes Way, Drouin, Victoria (thatveganhairdresser.com)
Publik Salon, 31 Emily Way, Varsity Lakes, Queensland (publik.com.au)
Chi Hair, 191 Canterbury Road, Victoria (chihair.com.au)

NEW ZEALAND

Earth Organic Hairdressing, 181 High Street, Christchurch (earthorganichairdressing.co.nz)
PETA-approved Shout Hair, 166 Richmond Road, Grey Lynn, Auckland (shouthair.co.nz)

BEAUTY

See the world
and explore
new places.

TRA

VEL

IN (KIND) STYLE

Aah, the dizzying magic of *le voyage*.

That buzzing moment of stepping onto a plane, train, or whatever your preferred method of transport may be, knowing that you're heading for an adventure. New discoveries. Territories unknown. Or, you know, just a really nice week of poolside relaxation.

Wherever you're heading, cruelty-free travel has never been easier—last time I got off a train at the Termini station in Rome, I found that one of the station cafés had a vegan sandwich, clearly labeled "vegan." Gone are the days when you'd have to pack your own meals for a long-haul flight; most airline companies now offer plant-based meals. Gone are the days when you couldn't enjoy a latte at the airport café because soy milk was nowhere to be found. And the days when all luggage was made from leather are definitely gone. In this chapter, we will explore the most chic ways to travel cruelty-free.

Keep in mind that wherever you are, it's crucial to avoid any entertainment that uses animals. Elephant and camel rides, swimming with dolphins, selfies with tigers, roadside zoos and animal circuses—all of these are likely to have taken the animals from their natural habitats and drugged or abused them to make them comply. Animals don't perform tricks for humans because they like it; they only do so because of the threat of what happens if they don't. So stick to entertainment featuring willing human performers only.

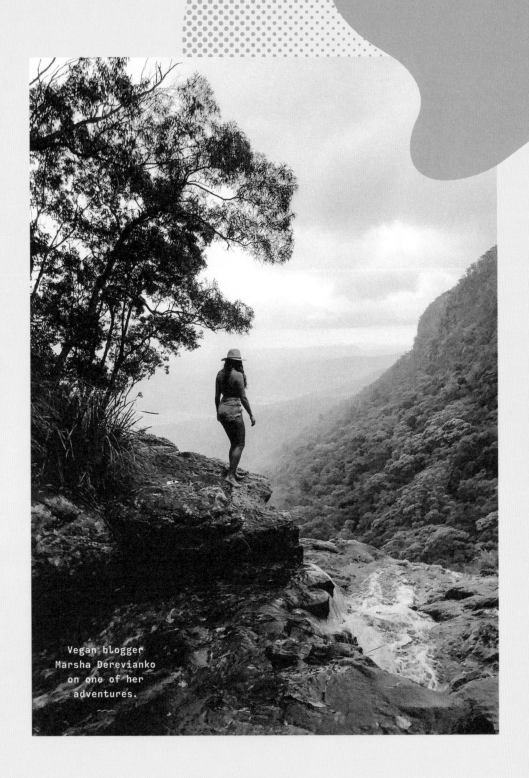

Vegan blogger
Marsha Derevianko
on one of her
adventures.

PLANNING AHEAD

To me, planning a trip is almost as exhilarating as the trip itself. Choosing a destination, booking the hotel (flicking through the pictures on hotel websites is addictive), writing the packing lists, packing—the joys of packing!—and, finally, carry-on in tow, setting off for the airport. Is there anything better?

Well, yes—a trip where you know your compassionate values won't leave you grazing on salad leaves for a week while your friends feast on exotic treats. Raise your hand if you've never been that person ordering a side salad while abroad, becoming an instant target for "poor you" looks from meat-devouring travel companions. I didn't think so. However, the key to not being that person lies in planning ahead. It can be as easy as finding the local vegan group in your destination and asking for advice (Google and Facebook are your friends here), but often the best weapon at your disposal is the HappyCow app and Happycow.net—a fantastic invention that will let you know exactly what vegan, vegetarian, and veggie-friendly places are to be found in your current location. It isn't completely exhaustive, but it offers a good overview. Another app, Veganagogo, helps you order your vegan meal in a variety of languages.

Secondly, if you're staying in a hotel, email them to ask about whether they cater to vegans. Make sure you explain what vegan means; once they know what you're asking for, they're better equipped to deal with your request. You might find yourself very surprised— many hotels, especially in tourist-friendly destinations, are getting more and more used to vegetarians and vegans. A tip: hit the buffets. Among the selection, there's bound to be at least something plant-based. I survived almost an entire vacation in Corfu by indulging in local delicacies at the hotel dinner buffet.

If you're renting an apartment with a kitchen—or Airbnb accommodation—there really are no excuses. Fruit, vegetables, nuts, and beans are readily available in every corner of the globe.

Best apps for vegan travelers

Before you next head out on the road, download these apps to make your vegan adventure even easier.

HappyCow

The obvious topper of this list is HappyCow—the app that tells you exactly how far you are from your nearest vegan eatery. Aside from listing all the vegan and vegetarian restaurants, it also tells you every place that has vegan options or is veggie-friendly. Lifesaver.

PlantEaters

This free app will tell you where to get vegan food abroad—and it also includes reviews from fellow plant-based travelers. Focusing on meals rather than restaurants, this is an app that will show you the way to many yummy dishes on the road.

AirVegan

Heading for the airport and not sure whether you should bring snacks? The answer to that is always yes, but just in case, download this app to see what vegan food offerings are available at the airport. The app has a color-rating system in which green means that vegan options abound, whereas red stands for scarce, in which case it's best to remember to BYOH (bring your own hummus).

Veganagogo

To ensure communication flows more smoothly, download this app, which features professionally translated sentences in over fifty languages, tailored to the vegan traveler. With questions like "Can you please show me which items on your menu contain no meat or animal products?" and "Is the chef able to make me a meal that contains no meat or animal products?" this app ensures that you will never be served a salad with grated cheese on top again.

Vegan Passport

This app was developed by The Vegan Society in order to make it easier for vegan travelers to order food abroad. Not only does the app feature translated sentences to communicate with 96 percent of the world's population, it also has handy drawings to show what vegans do and don't eat, and helps you book vegan meals with your airline. So many problems solved!

THE TASTIEST TRAVEL DESTINATIONS for vegans

Generally, vegan food can be found absolutely everywhere. For proof, see the blog *Veggsocial*, founded by activists Ryan Huling and Joel Bartlett, who posted photos of vegan dishes from every country in the world to prove that there are no excuses—you can take your vegan diet with you wherever you go. And that's really no wonder, since fruit, vegetables, pulses, and grains are available everywhere.

But, if you're anything like me, you enjoy a fine evening out at a restaurant every once in a while. Cooking is lovely, but many travelers don't have access to a kitchen (tip: get a room or house with one if you can), plus dining out is one of the luxuries of life—one that vegans don't have to miss out on at all. And when it comes to dining out, some places in the world are easier than others for plant-based travelers.

SYDNEY

Sydney offers a variety of options for the hungry vegan. Try authentic Italian pizza at Gigi's, indulge in burgers at Soul Burger, or get an ice cream at Gelato Blue. Sydney's first vegan pub, The Green Lion, is definitely on my must-try list. For some vegan health and beauty shopping, head to The Cruelty Free Shop: a 100 percent vegan store offering food, cosmetics, and household items such as cleaning products and candles.

TAIPEI

Taipei won the top spot on PETA Asia's 2017 list of the world's most vegan-friendly cities for gems such as Ooh Cha Cha, where you can find vegan versions of meaty burgers; Loving Hut, which offers everything from kimchi to cupcakes; and Soul R. Vegan Café, where plant-based gourmets can enjoy vegan steaks and faux prawns.

✕✕✕

Melbourne

Melbourne has almost one hundred vegan-friendly restaurants, according to HappyCow at the time of writing this book. Try Smith & Deli for a vegan poached egg (!), enjoy a vegan pizza at Red Sparrow Pizza, or tacos at Trippy Taco. Are you a health-food fan? Go wild with the deluxe smoothie selection at Matcha Mylkbar. If you, like me, are a huge fan of desserts, then Girls & Boys will be your new favorite: this takeout spot offers fudge bars, cakes, and ice cream. Bonus: it's right next to Vegie Bar, another plant-based hotspot.

✕✕✕

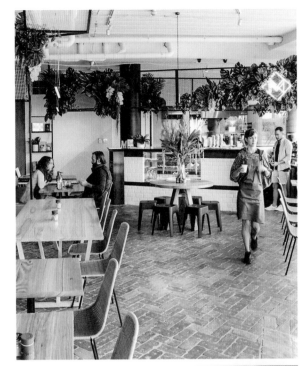

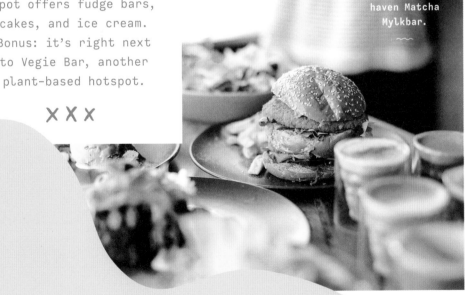

Melbourne vegan haven Matcha Mylkbar.

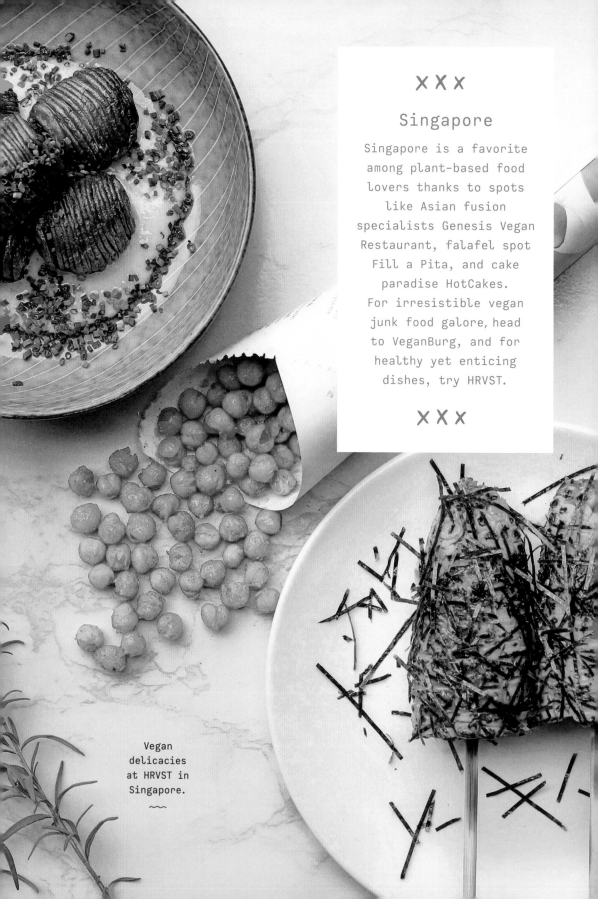

Singapore

Singapore is a favorite among plant-based food lovers thanks to spots like Asian fusion specialists Genesis Vegan Restaurant, falafel spot Fill a Pita, and cake paradise HotCakes. For irresistible vegan junk food galore, head to VeganBurg, and for healthy yet enticing dishes, try HRVST.

× × ×

Vegan delicacies at HRVST in Singapore.
~~~

LONDON

London is a mecca for vegan culinary exploration that never ends. During my four years of living in the English capital, I had the chance to sample so many indulgences—and there are so many left to try. Among the top contenders for best vegan eatery are comfort food spot Manna, gourmet burger paradise Mildreds, and innovative health-food haven Vantra. If you happen to be in the King's Cross area, stop by the all-vegan shop Vx for takeout, vegan snacks, and cakes.

BRIGHTON

Brighton is my current hometown, and it's the most vegan-friendly place I've ever been. It's not a huge city, so you can walk everywhere and can thus fit more eats into a single day—but it takes more than an entire vacation to explore all the plant-based delicacies this city has to offer. The United Kingdom's first 100 percent vegan pizzeria, Purezza, is just by the seafront, whereas the quirky shopping neighborhood The Lanes offers vegan junk food at Wai Kika Moo Kau, huge platefuls for £7 at Iydea, and vegan ice cream in unexpected flavors (dark chocolate and rose, anyone?) at Boho Gelato. For finer dining, head to Food for Friends or Terre à Terre—both vegetarian, but with lots of vegan options.

NEW YORK

New York has been considered one of the most vegan-friendly cities on the planet for a long time, and if you hear about a new vegan shop, restaurant, or fashion label popping up, you can bet that nine times out of ten, it will be here. Pioneering vegan brand VAUTE has their boutique here, and the city is a haven for delicious plant-based food, from the Impossible Burger (which looks and tastes exactly like meat) to mouthwatering doughnuts at Dun-Well.

LOS ANGELES

Los Angeles is the number-one spot for health-minded vegans, with a vast selection of plant-based options that are great for the mind, body, and spirit. Enjoy organic and seasonal meals at Café Gratitude, Mediterranean-inspired delights at Moby's restaurant Little Pine, and sophisticated deliciousness at Crossroads. If you're in the mood for shopping, don't miss Vegan Scene, a concept store in vibrant Venice Beach carrying men's and women's fashion, gifts, and accessories.

BERLIN

Berlin topped HappyCow's list of best destinations for vegan travelers in 2017. The German city is known as a plant-based paradise and boasts an entire area dedicated to vegetarian and vegan restaurants. From greasy burgers to raw gourmet cuisine, Berlin is the place to be if you're a vegan traveler. Places to try: superfood haven LAB Kitchen; mouthwatering bakery Cafe Velicious; and the entirely vegan supermarket Veganz, full of plant-based goodness.

If you're after more than just food, explore the vegan shopping at DearGoods, a fashion concept store offering fair-trade, organic, and vegan designs.

PARIS

Paris has recently upped the stakes in its plant-based offerings—in just a few years, it's gone from a relatively clueless place when it comes to anything meat-free to a culinary destination full of veggie delights. Visit the refined eatery Gentle Gourmet for creative dishes crafted from fresh and zesty ingredients, or why not try raw vegan dining at 42 Degrés? Relish the feeling of being able to eat everything on the menu at 100 percent vegan Café Ginger, then finish off with dessert at Patisserie V.

AMSTERDAM

Amsterdam was chosen as the most vegan-friendly city in Europe by vacation rental company Holidu in 2017. See just how creative plant-based dining can be at the Meatless District restaurant, sample eclectic international cuisine from all corners of the world at Jackson Dubois, and finish off with dessert at Koffie ende Koeck, an all-vegan cafe serving baked goods that will seriously tempt your taste buds. If you happen to be in town for Amsterdam Fashion Week, remember that it's one of the relatively few Fashion Weeks in the world that is 100 percent fur-free.

MILAN

Milan was not vegan-friendly at all when I lived there—but in the last few years, veggie food offerings have really blossomed in this northern Italian city. Grab a burger at one of Universo Vegano's locations, explore innovative vegetarian cuisine at Joia, or have the best tiramisu of your life at Alhambra Cafè. Bonus: you can now enjoy soy milk in your cappuccino at most of the city's cafes, which wasn't the case when I called this place home. Back then, some baristas didn't even know what soy milk was!

IN-FLIGHT SNACKING

Plane food has also had an upgrade since those "chicken or fish?" containers, with many major airlines now catering to vegans. You will probably need to call your airline in advance to order your meal, but a meal is likely to be available, and with a little bit of luck it will be tasty, too. Despite all this newfound abundance, I always bring snacks on flights. Nuts, fruit, and avocado sandwiches are easy to pack and make for great in-flight nibbles. If you're in the United Kingdom, check out the Graze box, a monthly subscription service that offers snacks—many of them vegan-friendly—in little plastic containers that are ridiculously easy to carry and can be delivered right to your home or office. Graze snacks are now available in British supermarkets as well. Another tip is Nakd bars and nibbles—they come in deviously delicious flavors (bakewell tart or salted caramel, anyone?) and contain nothing except dates, raisins, and other types of dried nuts and fruit. No sugar or any toxic nasties, just natural, vegan goodness.

AIRPORT SHOPPING

Airports have evolved into small shopping centres of their own, and we're not just talking about the duty-free shop—high-end boutiques stand side-by-side with casual cafes, and you can now buy anything from caviar to Victoria's Secret lingerie before you board your flight—or you could go for some cruelty-free makeup and that soy latte.

The best airports that cater for vegan needs are, unsurprisingly, in the United States. John F. Kennedy International, Newark Liberty International, and San Francisco International are among the leaders when it comes to offering vegan food on the go—sandwiches, wraps, snacks, and baked goods are just a sliver of what's on offer if you're lucky enough to have a layover in any of these hubs. In the United Kingdom, most large airports will have a Pret A Manger—the healthy fast-food chain with a gazillion veggie and vegan options. Beauty brand The Body Shop also sells its cruelty-free (and often vegan) cosmetics in many British airports. If you're at Stansted or Heathrow in London, or at the airport in Bristol, Belfast, or Edinburgh, check out Superdrug—a well-known British drugstore chain that carries several cruelty-free makeup brands, along with its own-name brand that's Leaping Bunny–approved and vegan. Many of their products come in travel sizes—a perfect way to pick up everything you need before it's time to board the plane.

PACK YOUR BAGS
ethical vegan luggage

A suitcase has quite a few responsibilities: not only is its job to contain your stuff but it also has to contain it securely and keep it safe from rain, wind, and dirt (if it wants to be a good suitcase), and be somewhat simple to transport—I remember the days when I first moved to Milan with a suitcase that didn't have wheels. Such a bad idea. Ideally, it should also look stylish. For cruelty-free travelers, there's yet another box to tick: it has to be leather-free. Luckily, many of the new travel companions are made from sturdy, high-tech, man-made materials (some of them recycled) that are free from leather and other animal-derived materials, and will make your journey stress-free as well as cruelty-free.

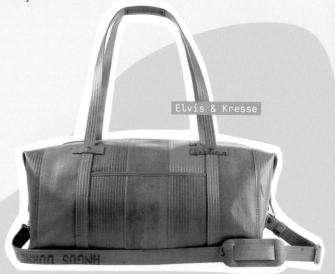

Elvis & Kresse

VEGAN STYLE

Some companies that are excelling in ethical luggage

Heys America

This travel expert company is home to the Eco Orbis, a suitcase made entirely from recycled plastic that would otherwise end up in a landfill. Durable, flexible, and stylish, the Eco Orbis is one sleek number.

Matt & Nat

If you're a longtime vegan shopper, you will already be familiar with Matt & Nat. If you're not, you're still guaranteed to have stumbled across them in this book. This Canadian label is a vegan fashion classic—and their elegant weekenders in muted colors are the mark of a stylish, compassionate traveler.

Elvis & Kresse

This brand is really something special. All their bags are made from reclaimed materials that would otherwise have gone to a landfill. They use recycled fire hoses (!) to create utility-chic overnight bags and duffel bags. A word of warning, though: some of the linings are made from parachute silk, so, as always, check the label.

Patagonia

If you're more of an outdoorsy travel type, Patagonia's sportswear-inspired suitcases might be more up your alley. The label promotes safe working conditions and fair labor practices for their workers, and you'll be happy to know that many of their vegan-friendly duffel bags and weekenders are made with recycled polyester.

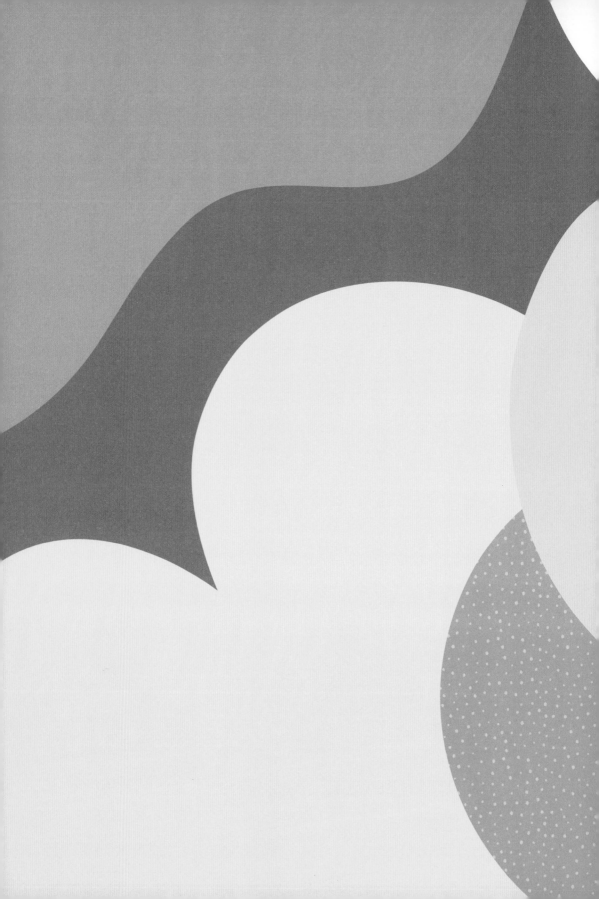

Wherever you're heading, cruelty-free travel has never been easier.

HOW TO PACK

Packing for a trip can be stressful, but getting all your vegan-friendly essentials ready for takeoff doesn't have to be a pain. Start with determining the items that will best suit not only the destination but also the purpose of the trip, and then choose the best luggage that will make traveling more effortless and pleasurable, leaving you to fully concentrate on your destination and experiences.

CITY BREAK
▽

get your bag from

Deux Lux

This ethical accessory brand specializes in vegan fashion with a whimsical twist. The Weekender range is comfortable and easy to match—and can even be monogrammed. The luxury.

don't forget to pack

A faux-leather jacket from New York City brand Dauntless. No one will be able to tell that you aren't wearing real leather—that's how authentic these jackets look, without any of the cruelty of the real deal.

travel in

A pair of Monkee Genes. Made in England from organic cotton, all Monkee styles carry the PETA-approved vegan logo.

BEACH VOYAGE
▽

get your bag from

Kayu

This is not a 100 percent vegan brand, but environmentally sustainable label Kayu does offer many amazing vegan beach options, some of which are made with natural seagrass.

don't forget to pack

A bikini from Swoon Swimwear. The feel-good style of these bikinis is as uplifting as the fact that they're all locally produced in the United States and free from child labor.

travel with

An eye-catching luggage tag from vegan brand Harveys.

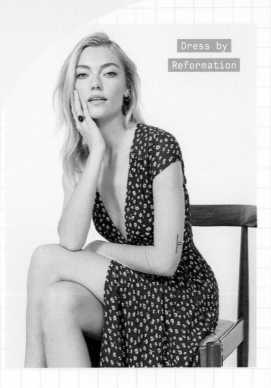

Dress by
Reformation

WINTER ESCAPE

get your bag from

Thamon

Pack your essentials in a backpack
from this London label that offers
accessories made from leaves.
Thamon also offers cork bags for
both men and women.

don't forget to pack

A wool-free scarf from ethical
marketplace Bead & Reel. They come in
a variety of designs, don't sting or itch,
and are, of course, cruelty-free and
ethically produced. Win.

travel with

A chunky cable knit from VAUTE.
Airports can get chilly,
so stay toasty with this ethical,
locally produced, vegan range of
stylish knitwear.

ROMANTIC GETAWAY

get your bag from

Alexandra K

From sleek black to rich jewel hues,
this cruelty-free Polish brand offers
a range of travel accessories that
will turn heads.

don't forget to pack

A date dress from possibly the coolest
ethical brand in existence: Reformation.

travel with

Some comfortable yet stylish ankle
boots from French vegan shoe brand
By Blanch.

MARSHA DEREVIANKO

LUXURY VEGAN TRAVEL BLOGGER

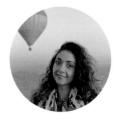

"I spend a lot of my life searching for food."

She wanted to see the world, so she started a luxury travel blog. Only hitch? She's vegan. But her plant-based lifestyle has only worked to Marsha Derevianko's advantage; her blog *World Within Her* has won awards and taken her around the globe. Here are her best tips for vegan travelers:

None of my previous jobs, from personal shopping to sales, were fulfilling for me. I always knew that I wanted to work for myself and be an entrepreneur. My biggest passion is travel, so after thinking about what I could do that would let me travel the world, starting a blog seemed like a good idea, as it would allow me to work from anywhere in the world. I had an epic trip to Thailand that my then-boyfriend planned, so I documented our days as an online diary for my friends and family to keep track of our shenanigans, and this is how *World Within Her* started.

I spend a lot of my life searching for food. I think one of the biggest

difficulties is traveling to countries who think being a veggie means you still eat fish; #lestruggleisreal. In the past, when I found myself in places where the variety of vegan foods was limited, I ended up eating a lot of bread, which I don't really like to do. I now make sure I have superfood snacks with me when I travel, as well as multivitamins to get all my necessary goodies in. I request to have a superfood smoothie in the mornings from my hotel, or I add the superfoods to my breakfast so at least that way I get a kickstart to days full of bread, bland salads, and oily vegetable casseroles.

Among the destinations that blew my mind for catering exceptionally well to plant-based foodies, Prague stood out. I was astonished at how vegan-friendly it was, how many vegan restaurants they had, and how delicious the food was. Considering it's an Eastern European country with a general diet that consists largely of red meat, potatoes, and weird parts of animals, the vegan offerings were really amazing.

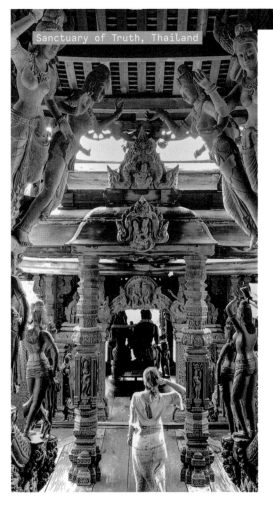

Sanctuary of Truth, Thailand

Marsha's tips for cruelty-free travelers

Make sure you have snacks or food when you land at your destination.

~~~

Always bring your superfoods and multivitamins to make sure that, regardless of what you eat locally, you're getting enough nutrients.

~~~

Download the HappyCow app, as it's actually a lifesaver, then search out all the nearby places.

~~~

Read blogs about recommended vegan spots in the place you're visiting.

Being a vegan blogger has allowed me to meet the most revolutionary vegan chefs whose food is more of an experience than a meal. The most memorable vegan food I have had to date has been at Joia in Milan. Pietro Leemann takes you on a journey with each ingredient, and you can just taste the love in his masterpieces. Incredible!

My second-most memorable vegan trip has been to Miami; the vegan scene there is booming, and I was blown away by Plant Food + Wine and praise what Matthew Kenney is doing. He's another foodie extraordinaire whose presentation, blends of ingredients, and use of color are second to none.

BEAUTY BITS AND PIECES TO LOOK FRESH EN ROUTE

Airport shopping is more varied and multifaceted than ever before, so finding vegan-friendly beauty products before takeoff is easy. Look for these skin and hair helpers for a touch-up prior to landing.

HAND CREAM

•

Pacifica hand cream
Aside from the addictive scents (Pacifica is also a major player in the vegan perfume arena), these easy-to-carry creams are also moisturizing and softening, guaranteeing your hands will look and feel amazing when you land at your destination—even if it's freezing cold.

HAND SANITIZER

•

The Body Shop Satsuma Antibacterial Hand Sanitizer
Before you indulge in some luxurious hand cream, use some of this to freshen up. Forget that clinical smell; this stuff has a deliciously fruit-flavored scent.

LIP BALM

•

Hurraw! lip balm
Do not be a victim of chapped lips. Pick up one of these organic babies that has mega-moisturizing properties and comes in a range of delicious flavors.

DRY SHAMPOO

•

Batiste dry shampoo
This super-cheap hair helper comes in a variety of scents (my favorite is Tropical) and is an ideal helping hand against limp, flat "plane hair." Just turn your head upside-down, give it a few spritzes, tousle with your hands, and enjoy wonderfully messy, voluminous locks.

EYE DROPS

•

Superdrug moisturizing eye drops
If you're a contact-lens wearer like me (and even if you aren't), plane air wreaks havoc with your eyes, making them dry and itchy. Combat this with Superdrug's tiny little bottle of drops, which won't even leave your mascara smudged. Job done.

WHERE TO SHOP VEGAN FASHION ABROAD
international fashion directory

The best in vegan shopping is still to be found online—we are in the digital age, after all—but as interest in vegan living grows, so does the presence of brick-and-mortar shops around the globe offering vegan clothing and accessories. Find these on your next trip and enjoy the luxury of walking around in a shop and knowing that you can try on everything, because every item is 100 percent cruelty-free.

BERLIN/MUNICH/ AUGSBURG

DearGoods
Featuring womenswear, menswear, accessories, and lifestyle items, this ethical fashion boutique offers items that are sustainably produced with attention to workers' rights. Brands they carry include Matt & Nat, Miss Green, and Komodo, and their overall vibe is "hip Berlin girl or guy," which is exactly the look you want to take home when shopping in this impossibly cool city.
Find it here: the brand has three Munich locations, one in Berlin, and one in Augsburg.

GOTHENBURG

T H R I V E
The charming city of Gothenburg is a vegan mecca, and we're not just talking food: vegan shopping has never looked as good as it does at T H R I V E—a haven for all things ethical and sustainable. Founded by an entrepreneur and a renowned fashion photographer who wanted to bring a kinder edge to fashion, the shop offers clothing by People Tree, Armed Angels, and Bourgeois Boheme, among others, and also has a well-stocked online boutique.
Find it here: Södra Allégatan 11, Gothenburg

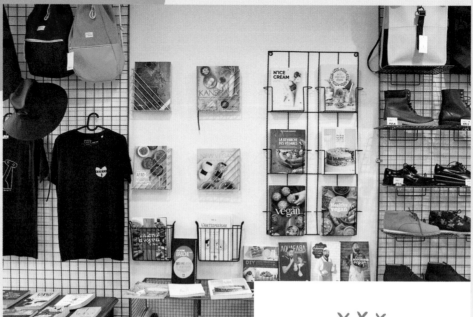

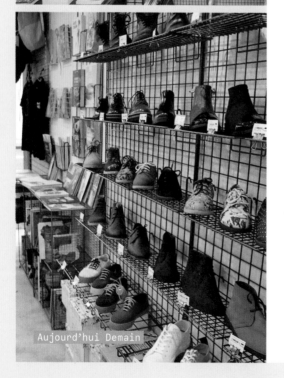

Aujourd'hui Demain

✕ ✕ ✕

PARIS

▽

Aujourd'hui Demain

This concept store has managed to merge Parisian chic with vegan ethics—and their contemporary aesthetic is cool enough to catch the eye of non-vegans as well. Offering food, fashion, cosmetics, and pet products, this shop is everything a vegan in Paris can dream of. **Find it here: 42 Rue de Chemin Vert, Paris**

✕ ✕ ✕

LOS ANGELES

▽

Vegan Scene

This concept store in Los Angeles is described by its founder, Amy Rebecca Wilde, as "Studio 54 with more quinoa" (for more from Amy, see chapter 7, page 160). A favorite of vegan celebs Mayim Bialik and Alicia Silverstone, who have both tweeted about this place, Vegan Scene also has two of its own vegan fashion ranges, Legends & Vibes and Rebelives.

Find it here: 4051 Lincoln Boulevard, Los Angeles

MELBOURNE

▽

Vegan Style

Focusing on vegan fashion exclusively, this Australian boutique offers men's, women's, and unisex shoes and accessories, and several cosmetics ranges as well. This is the go-to place for a variety of leather-free shoes and bags, and if you can't get to Melbourne, you can shop their vast collection online.

Find it here: 345 Brunswick Street, Fitzroy, Melbourne

LONDON

The Third Estate

Of course, London, the ultimate "what's-new-in-fashion" city, had to have a vegan fashion boutique. Camden's The Third Estate is a shoe-focused shop, but you can also find bags and other men's and women's accessories here. Brands like Will's London, Matt & Nat, and Tivydale are just a few of the reasons to visit this shop; the vibrant atmosphere of Camden is another.

Find it here: 27 Brecknock Road, London

STOCKHOLM

Green Laces

Another Swedish shop, and this one is also focused on shoes. Veja, Teva, and Camminaleggero are just a few brands carried by this ethical shop, which also offers gorgeous bags from brands like Matt & Nat and Sanquist. If you're going to explore the Scandi-chic scene, don't forget to stop here.

Find it here: Hökens Gata 7, Stockholm

MY LATEST MEDITERRANEAN TRIPS
in order of vegan friendliness

Despite growing up in Sweden and currently living in the United Kingdom, I believe that I am Mediterranean at heart. I lived in Italy for six years, and it remains my favorite southern European travel destination, but most Mediterranean countries have really stepped up their game in terms of vegan-friendliness. Check this mini-guide before booking your next flight.

ITALY

Recent spikes in vegan living in Italy have fostered an amazing rise in plant-based options. Italian cuisine is naturally quite rich in vegan foods—I'm talking countless pasta dishes with vegetable sauces, meat-free pizza, and more—but big cities are now aware of veganism and cater to it with surprising creativity and flair. Restaurants to visit in Milan include Alhambra, Joia, and fast-food chain Universo Vegano (where I had my first-ever kebab). In the south, Naples proved to be an unexpected vegan paradise: enjoy vegan delicacies at Sbuccia e Bevi and 'O Grin, but also don't miss the vegan tofu mozzarella Margherita at Sorbillo, or head to legendary L'antica Pizzeria da Michele for a marinara—the original pizza.

PORTUGAL

My first-ever visit to Portugal in 2016 to review vegan-friendly Boutique Hotel Vivenda Miranda in Lagos showed me just how vegan-friendly this country can be. Aside from a fantastic vegan dinner at the hotel, I worried about finding plant-based options in the tiny seaside town of Lagos. Luckily, I was wrong: this Mediterranean town offered cafés that unexpectedly featured both seitan roast and a tofu curry.

SPAIN

If you're visiting Barcelona, you're in luck—the city actually has a program to promote plant-based living and declared itself a "vegetarian-friendly city" in 2015. Bigger Spanish cities are often familiar with veganism and vegetarianism, but even smaller towns can be good at offering meat-free options: I survived on veggie paella and grilled vegetables (with the added protein of tins of beans in my hotel room) during my holiday to the Costa Brava. I'm not usually a fan of potatoes (shock, horror!), but with the lack of other options, can be convinced to try patatas bravas; everything tastes better fried.

GREECE

Whereas meat and fish still largely rule the menus, Greek food does have some true delights for vegans. Try some dolmadakia—rice wrapped in vine leaves, which is one of my favorite dishes on the planet. Tip: check the starters and side dishes on the menu when out in Greece. You can often find exceptionally made bean dishes and eggplant salads, which will truly delight your palate. Supermarkets also provide good selections.

MALTA

And here we enter challenging territory. While Malta is absolutely stunning, the food is somewhat disappointing. Despite 37°C (98°F) heat, most of the food on offer during my holiday was fried and heavy: potatoes and rabbit (a traditional dish) or other heavily cooked dishes, which were better suited to chilly winter days. Anything even remotely healthy was difficult to find, but my struggles were all repaid at the fantastic Sammy's by Culinary Forward Malta in Xemxija: a 100 percent vegan menu with amazing, locally grown produce. So, as you see, vegan delights are to be found even where you least expect them.

ONES TO WATCH

Nine designers who are shaping the future of fashion.

THE STYLE CHANGEMAKERS

As interest for ethical and compassionate living grows, cruelty-free fashion is becoming more refined.

Brands are more trend-sensitive and care about catering not only to a vegan community but also to a more fashion-conscious client, without ever compromising on their values. Experimenting with natural materials like cork, recycled fabrics, and innovative textiles is second nature to the designers of these new wardrobe must-haves—and for the multibrand retailers hand-picking the selection of fashion to appear in their sleek (online as well as bricks-and-mortar) shops, innovation is key. That's why compassionate fashion is moving from a niche concept to a cool, hip person's value of choice.

Concern for animals isn't the only factor these people feel strongly about. Human rights, eco-friendly materials, and fair trade are all high on their list of priorities, making them all-around ethical powerhouses capable of transforming not only wardrobes but entire lifestyles. As transparency becomes more and more of a hot topic, and more customers want to know where their clothes came from, these new designers and retailers can proudly talk in detail about their supply chains, their materials, and #whomadetheirclothes—and this level of consciousness and awareness is what will make the fashion industry of the future. Gone are the days when status and ostentation were "it." Now, in order to have "it," you must not only be stylish but also sustainable.

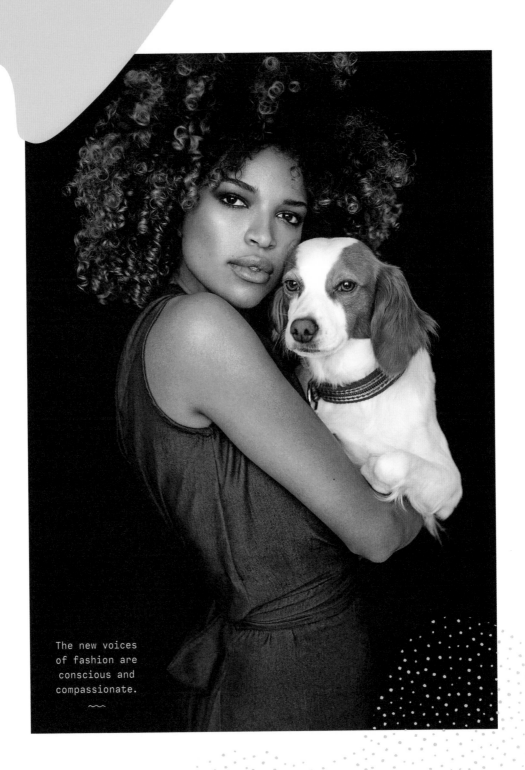

The new voices
of fashion are
conscious and
compassionate.

157

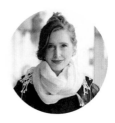

SICA SCHMITZ

FOUNDER OF BEAD & REEL

"I'm very excited and optimistic about the future of fashion."

Offering a curated selection of over sixty independent designers, online boutique Bead & Reel focuses on ethical values such as veganism and also fair trade, locally made in the United States, organic, and female-founded businesses. The brand was founded by former Hollywood costume designer Sica Schmitz in Los Angeles. She told me a bit about how she got started:

I studied fashion design and, through a series of unexpected and yet fortunate events, I ended up going into costume design for film and television, which I did for many years, everywhere from Hollywood to Ireland.

I've always loved fashion and storytelling, and founding Bead & Reel was my way of bringing them together in a very meaningful way. After the Rana Plaza factory collapse in Bangladesh in 2013 (which killed over 1,100 garment workers), I became

increasingly interested in fair-trade fashion. The catalyst for Bead & Reel was one afternoon that I spent searching for shoes that were both vegan and ethically made, and I was shocked at how difficult it was to find something that took animals and people into equal consideration. It took extensive research to finally find a pair that was both ethically and aesthetically pleasing, and I wondered why there wasn't just somewhere that you could shop that made it easier for busy people like me to shop their values without spending hours digging around online. Since something like that didn't yet exist, I decided to create it. I ended up leaving my job on a TV show I had been working on for several years and launched Bead & Reel in 2014.

I hold my designers to a very high standard. All the products we carry at Bead & Reel are vegan (of course) and, beyond that, they must be made under ethical and legal manufacturing standards (our criteria are based on the International Organization for Standardization Social Responsibility standards and World Fair Trade Organization fair-trade principles, among other guidelines). Whenever possible, I try to choose eco-friendly materials (organic, recycled, up-cycled), and I emphasize female-founded businesses; if we want to support women, we have to support women-owned companies.

There are fifteen different ethical criteria that I identify at Bead & Reel, and I try to find brands and products that meet as many of these as possible. Beyond these, the garments have to be wearable. I've styled and dressed hundreds (if not thousands) of women throughout my career, and it's important for me to carry styles that will make women feel beautiful and comfortable.

The final criterion is being an ethical company—by that, I mean they have to actually care about their customers, care about quality, and care about creating a positive impact on the world. Making vegan, fair-trade, and/or organic fashion does not necessarily mean that a company is ethical (unfortunately there are a lot of very disappointing companies who are taking advantage of buzzwords to drive sales while cutting a lot of important corners), and I'm so proud of having personal relationships with every brand I carry.

I don't think I've found being an ethical business owner any more challenging than being a traditional business owner. Being a business owner is just difficult in general. I actually think operating under a strong set of values makes it easier in some ways, as it clarifies my options and direction. I could write far too much about the challenges of starting a business, growing a business, and all the hard lessons I've learned along the way, but I think having very clear ethics, nurturing my intuition, and having an incredibly supportive network of people in my life make the daily obstacles very manageable.

I'm very excited and optimistic about the future of fashion. I think, realistically, the industry is going to have to shift more toward sustainable production. Our planet simply cannot keep up with the way we're making things and tossing things. And I definitely see a growing number of people insisting on vegan fashion and fair-trade fashion, and I think fashion brands are going to start moving in that direction in order to stay competitive. I hope the future of ethical fashion encompasses the protection of all that are vulnerable—people, animals, and the environment—and not just favors one or two.

Shop Bead & Reel at beadandreel.com.

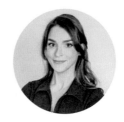

AMY REBECCA WILDE

ENTREPRENEUR BEHIND
VEGAN SCENE

"The evolution of vegan fashion is about getting people to understand that veganism is more than just a diet."

I personally credit Amy with having motivated me to go vegan. Her wonderful Instagram account @vegansofig opened my eyes to how easy it could be to adopt this lifestyle. After starting local activist group Fur Free LA, which helped convince boutiques such as Intermix and Planet Blue to stop selling fur, Amy started the vegan boutique and event space Vegan Scene in Los Angeles. Amy explains how she was destined to be vegan from a young age:

I went vegetarian at seven years old, and vegan at fifteen. I have always described myself as a "quirky vegan with a shopping problem," and one of my favorite stores has always been Planet Blue in Los Angeles. So when I noticed that they sold fur, I decided to do something about it—I've always found fur to be such an unnecessary opulence. I had just returned to Los Angeles after living in Italy, and winters here are so warm that there seemed to be even less need for fur. So I decided to protest outside the store—just me and my dog, Louie—handing out flyers to passersby. People stopped, asked questions, showed interest, so I set up Facebook events for more protests, and more people showed up and joined me each time. That's how my first activist project, Fur Free LA, got started. We always made sure we looked stylish and fashionable, so the stores would know they would lose actual customers over the decision to sell fur. And Planet Blue did go fur-free—it turned out that they didn't know about the cruelty of fur. That's how I realized that I wanted to focus on educating people. I felt quite lonely as a vegan, as I didn't know many other vegans. In an attempt to reach out to people, I set up

@vegansofig, an Instagram account where I shared information on why and how to go vegan.

After the @vegansofig account got a bit of traction, I started traveling around the country organizing vegan meetups. When I was doing this, I realized that there was a need for an event space for vegans, so I started my own. It was important for me to have the word "vegan" in the name—and I would say that this hasn't hurt the business at all, despite the fact that most of our clients are omnivores. The fashion boutique side of the business took off, and we realized that we needed to start our own line to offer people a line of high-end looks along with more basic designs. What's keeping some people from transitioning to a vegan lifestyle is the perception that it's limiting and difficult, so we want to offer people a fashionable choice without being preachy.

We recently launched two own-brand clothing lines, Legends & Vibes and Rebelives. It's easy for vegan fashion to be expensive, but by taking control of our own designs, we ensure everything is vegan and locally produced—and reasonably priced. We wanted to create a spectrum of designs and offer both basics and more glamorous pieces that you can feel amazing in, and that meet every one of our ethical checkpoints.

Aside from educating and explaining to vendors what vegan means, most of the challenges are connected to running a business, rather than an ethical business. You need a strong team with you, and I've been lucky to have people on board who work hard to revolutionize fashion and bring vegan fashion to the mainstream.

Issues such as climate change, global warming, and workers' rights have ignited conversations within the fashion industry.

For me, the evolution of vegan fashion is largely about getting people to understand that veganism is more than just a diet. Vegan living has really taken off in the last few years, and people are connecting with it, but the fashion side still has a way to go. Issues such as climate change, global warming, and workers' rights have ignited conversations within the fashion industry, and these things have become talking points for a reason. We really need to show that there is a market for animal-free fashion.

Visit Vegan Scene at veganscene.com or at 4051 Lincoln Boulevard, Los Angeles, California.

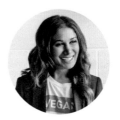

*BLOGGER TURNED
VEGAN SHOE DESIGNER*

"I saw a gap in the market for luxury vegan shoes."

As one of the first vegan fashion bloggers, Australian Nadhisha inspired thousands of people online every day to dress cruelty-free, but recently she decided to take her passion for style one step further by creating vegan footwear. Her brand, Huntd, launched with just a few pump designs, but is growing and expanding, offering luxury-loving customers high-end vegan designs. Nadhisha told me a bit about the evolution of her business:

I have a background in graphic design with a Bachelors Degree in Design and Visual Communications. Realizing that graphic design, photography, and other forms of visual communication were not for me when choosing a career path, I worked in market research for four years before leaving because I felt unfulfilled. I wanted to follow my passion for fashion in some way, but had no

official qualifications, and therefore turned my focus to creating a blog. At this time, it had been a few years since I had quit buying fashion items made from animal skins, and I had become quite good at finding vegan designer products. I wanted to share my research with others, and that's how my vegan fashion blog *Huntd* was created.

When I stopped buying non-vegan fashion, I definitely saw the gap in the market for luxury vegan products. Sure, you could go to any ordinary clothing store and find a huge variety of cheap vegan options, but there was a lack of well-designed and well-produced brands that were on-trend and ethical. I found that there were many well-made, high-end vegan brands, but not many had items that were my style. I always knew from a young age that I wanted to own my own business (in high school I always said I wanted to be a shoe designer), so I began to research starting my own label. I began by designing bags but really struggled, so I turned my focus to a core collection of shoes—shoes that every woman should have in her wardrobe—and Huntd was born.

I started my fashion journey back in 2015, and, since then, the vegan fashion scene has evolved in many ways. Firstly, I think people are starting to expect vegan fashion brands to also be ethical and transparent in their processes. I think the natural step for people who have become vegan is to then start to care for the environment and the people who manufacture the items. I personally think this is wonderful and have worked hard to ensure my brand is as ethical and transparent as possible. There are definitely many ways we can improve, and that's a promise I make to my customers—to ensure that my brand continues to find better alternatives and to keep improving.

I also think vegan fashion has evolved with fashion itself. Thanks to new companies and vegan fashion bloggers, animal-free fashion is no longer regarded as only for "hippies" or as being devoid of style and taste. There's a strong army of vegan fashion bloggers around the world showcasing looks that rival their non-vegan counterparts. We're showing the world that you do not need to sacrifice style in order to care for the animals and the planet. Vegan style can definitely be on-trend, luxurious, and fashion-forward.

I think when you're a new designer, you feel like people are scrutinizing every aspect of your business. I felt like people were expecting my products to be vegan, ethical, eco-friendly, charitable, and not made with profit in mind. I definitely felt the pressure of people asking questions and having expectations, such as why my brand only catered to vegans, why my shoes didn't have a range of nudes for every skin type, why my shoes were priced as they were, and so on. Before I felt all the pressure of having to be vegan-friendly, gender-friendly, skin tone-friendly, eco-friendly, etc., I had to refocus and tell myself that my three main objectives were to be kind to animals, the environment, and the people who made the shoes.

Being a new designer also means I work completely alone with no help. I do everything from the first designs to marketing, packaging, and customer service. At times, I feel overwhelmed when people place the same expectations on me thay they would on an established business with many more followers, but then I remember that it's a compliment that people expect so much, and I give my all to make my customers happy. I do hope one day that I can hire a team to help run the business. That is definitely a goal of mine.

See more from Huntd at huntd.com.au.

PATRICK DINKFELD

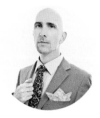

FOUNDER OF LOVELIGHT MODELS

"We must not let the race for wealth turn the ethical and conscious movement into yet another cheap fast-fashion trend."

A modeling agency focused entirely on vegan models sounds like a dream—but it's a reality thanks to visual artist and entrepreneur Patrick Dinkfeld, who has made it his mission to help ethically minded companies find models who mirror their values. He works with models in the United States, Australia, and Europe who share his vegan and compassionate ethical stance:

I've always been an artist, playing music, painting, and drawing, but it wasn't until college that I started exploring visual art through photography, film, and video. I spent the early years of my graphic-design career creating motion-graphics and digital video projects for corporate clients around the world, and eventually found myself gravitating toward fine art and fashion photography.

During my time experimenting with photography, I also started a deep and profoundly transformative meditation practice. Through my studies and meditation, I came to a point where it was important for me to align every aspect of my existence with my meditative and experiential existence.

As I looked to my art, I noticed I had fallen out of love with my photography. I realized I could no longer work with just any random model. Sometimes models would show up for a shoot and their energy would be really toxic, negative, or simply so extremely different from my own that I found myself thinking, "I don't want to spend all day with this person. I can't make *art* of this person." So, I started hand-picking my models based on their entire being. I started selecting my muses based on their energy as a being and not only on their physical appearance.

This immediately brought my experience of the art-making process into alignment with everything else I was working on with my meditation practice and my life. After a few years of shooting with models whose vibration and energy brought added depth to our shoots, I had a fairly good network of talent and friends who really inspired me in these ways. So, I thought, "I wonder if anyone else would care about this like I do?" And from that, I decided to put together a group of talent with this focus in mind, to see what kind of inspiring change we might be able to bring to the world through our creative endeavors. This moment of revelation was about two years ago.

At first, it was about five of my friends—models I had worked with previously and had great success with, and who also shared a passion for conscious living as well as a desire to bring more depth to their art. The early months were mostly me trying to figure out what this agency could truly be and how we might actually go about explaining the idea to the world. Eventually, I started expanding the recruiting and talent search and found some absolutely captivating and inspiring souls who shared my desires.

The agency quickly grew into something that was clearly going to be much bigger. I realized that we had the opportunity to change what it meant to be a model or a celebrity. We had the opportunity to create influencers with depth, and actually seek to make this planet a better place.

We now have over seventy models across the United States, Australia, and Western Europe. And we are about to begin producing our own content in an effort to inspire, entertain, and educate consumers on a variety of conscious ideas, starting with veganism, sustainable fashion, and conscious living.

To me, living ethically and operating an ethical business means living life better than I did in the past. Beyond that, I hope to inspire others to join the conversation and encourage them to expand on their idea of what is possible and within their reach.

In the world of ethical fashion, we have two roles to play in reevaluating our culture of consumption. First, we must play the role of creative artist and inspiring leader. We show people what is possible when we act ethically and consciously. Then, as the world shifts toward a more conscious way of living and consuming, we must provide the resources and products, ensuring integrity always remains at the core. We must not let the race for wealth turn the ethical and conscious movement into yet another cheap fast-fashion trend.

Check out Lovelight Models at LovelightModels.com.

JULIA KOCH

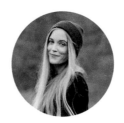

*COFOUNDER OF
VEGAN GOOD LIFE
MAGAZINE*

"I knew that Vegan Good Life was a product that could change people's perspectives on veganism, and that I was in a position to really make that happen."

Former model Julia decided to diversify into creating a magazine that reflected her vegan values. Born as a German counterculture publication, *Vegan Good Life* is now published in two languages and is a hit with hipster vegans around Europe. Julia told me a bit about how it all started:

I was modeling in Milan, London, and New York for several years when I decided to pack up all my things and move back to my hometown to study agricultural science. I loved my job and I earned a ridiculous amount of money, but I wasn't happy at all. I missed my friends and family but, more importantly, at some point, I realized that fashion isn't at all about freedom, art, and design.

It's more about being better, richer, and more sophisticated than others. The only reason that most fashion designers and brands are successful is that they profit from horrible production and labor conditions and create an artificial desire to follow a certain trend. I do think that fashion is a tool to express yourself and to diversify from others, but what a lot of people don't realize is that their clothes had a life before they were hung in their closet.

After university, I worked for various communication agencies as a journalist until I finally found my way back into the fashion business about six years ago. Since my early twenties, I've worked for different vegan and sustainable fashion brands and retailers, and cofounded a vegan fashion blog and international print magazine. Since 2015, I have been an author for German *Vogue*'s partner blog *This is Jane Wayne.* (I currently live and work in Berlin.)

I always wished for a coffee-table magazine that not only covered all things beautiful and vegan in fashion, art, travel, and design but also had a high-end look and feel.

What a lot of people don't realize is that their clothes had a life before they were hung in their closet.

There were a few magazines on the international market that I like, but I couldn't identify with them. I already knew a lot about the horrible treatment of animals and the immense effect on the planet caused by the production of animal food and derivatives, and I really didn't want to engage with yet another publication that was propped up by it. What I was looking for was a positive, modern, and artful alternative about vegan living that I'd be happy to have in my home and show to my friends. My cofounder, Eric Mirbach, and I successfully started a blog with this approach about two years before the first issue of *Vegan Good Life* came out, and, after a few months, we had so many visitors to our website that we instantly knew we were on to something.

To be honest, I had no idea what I had gotten myself into when I decided to launch a bilingual and international print magazine. I didn't have any money, I was barely educated in distribution and economics, and I had no idea where to start. The only thing I had more than enough of was passion and the will to really make a difference for animals. I knew that *Vegan Good Life* was a product that could change people's perspectives on veganism and animal cruelty, and that I was in a position to really make that happen. I had a lot of experience in journalism, marketing, and fashion, and Eric is not only a great writer and photographer but also very talented in design and layout. The most amazing moment, however, was when we finally held our very first, freshly printed issue in our hands. I remember being so scared to look through the pages to find typos or any major layout mistakes that it took me a couple of minutes to finally look at the product I had worked so hard for. And, big surprise, of course we found a typo on the first page, in our editorial headline. But we survived.

Explore *Vegan Good Life* at vegan-good-life.com.

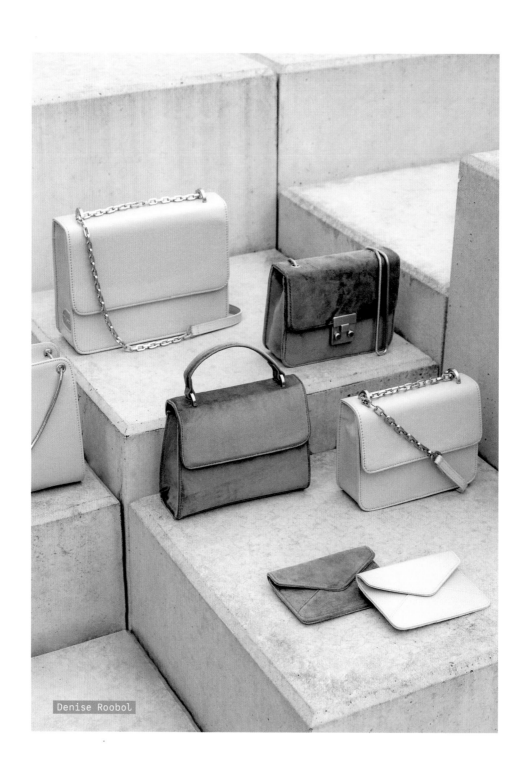

Denise Roobol

DENISE ROOBOL

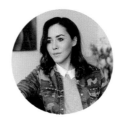

FOUNDER OF DENISE ROOBOL HANDBAGS

"I wanted to inspire people by showing that accessories can be vegan-friendly with a minimalistic and functional design."

Clean lines, stark silhouettes, and a minimalist aesthetic separate Denise Roobol's cruelty-free handbag brand from her competition. The Dutch designer's sleek and versatile designs are managing to entice non-vegans as well as remaining a favorite of the already converted.

I studied at the Willem de Kooning Academy of Lifestyle and Design in the Netherlands, and gradually went vegan after my eighteenth birthday.

I decided to start a vegan brand myself. I wanted to create something new in order to inspire people by showing them that fashion accessories can be vegan-friendly with minimalistic and functional design.

In the beginning, fashion boutiques weren't very open-minded about vegan products. In the Netherlands I have seen a big change, with vegan hotspots popping up everywhere in the big cities in the last two to three years.

To sell products to non-vegans is sometimes a big challenge, but my job and passion is to inform both vegans and non-vegans about the benefits of cruelty-free fashion. Sometimes it's about opening up the mind of a non-vegan, and I believe our success in doing this is that we don't scream "this is a vegan brand." Instead, our priority is to inspire and simply show that the product is vegan, to attract people to the design before the ethics.

I have to say that, in the last couple of years in particular, people have come around to the idea that vegans and vegetarians aren't the stereotype of fifteen years ago, and that's a great change.

Get one of Denise's bags at deniseroobol.com.

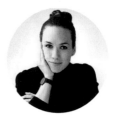

CAYLA MACKEY

COFOUNDER OF UNICORN GOODS

"In the future, 'ethical' will mean 'vegan,' as using animals for human consumption will be illegal."

Featuring an endless supply of men's, women's, and children's vegan fashion, as well as lifestyle and food items, Unicorn Goods is the biggest online catalogue for vegan style. The site's cofounder, Cayla Mackey, is a champion of female entrepreneurship and is a serial vegan entrepreneur:

Before cofounding Unicorn Goods with my partner, Dave Pittman, I had collaborated with him on several other businesses. We started a print and online magazine called *Native*, and a vegetarian breakfast taco bike called Taco Bike. I learned a lot about what it takes to run a successful ethical business by doing sales and operations for the various small startups that we co-owned. As our ethics evolved and we both became vegan, we launched Unicorn Goods to help people buy vegan products.

I first tried to buy a pair of non-leather shoes in 2014, and started to keep a spreadsheet of my options. I realized, through many failed purchases, that many companies didn't even know what was in their products, and that there wasn't an easy way to find vegan products. My partner and I soon realized that there was an opportunity to share the information I had amassed to help others locate vegan products, and we turned the spreadsheet into a website in December 2014. This was the culmination of our lives as vegetarians, as we realized that all the products we previously favored contributed to an industry we no longer wanted to be a part of on any level.

We are constantly researching vegan brands for Unicorn Goods. We have a database of hundreds of companies that we're already working with or that we want to work with. We vet all of these companies for holistic ethics and prioritize 100 percent vegan brands,

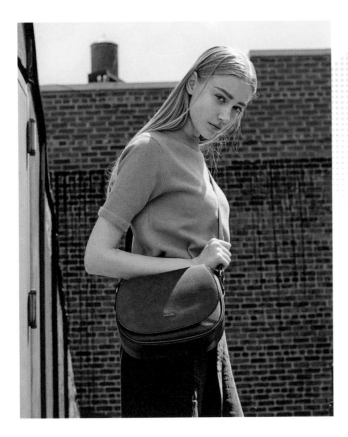

Unicorn Goods features fashion from brands who respect animals and the planet, such as this Angela Roi bag.

fair trade–certified companies, 1 percent for the Planet–certified companies, and companies that have a clear commitment to sustainability and transparent supply chains.

We had never launched a web-based business before, and the learning curve was very steep, especially with respect to the financial aspects of online marketing and e-commerce. I studied these areas until I understood them well enough to build our business model on them and continued to develop my

coding skills so that I could have a deeper understanding of our platform as it continued to grow and develop.

In the future, I believe that all products will be vegan, because it will be illegal to use animals for any kind of human consumption. The word "ethical" will be synonymous with "vegan," and we are excited to be on the crest of that wave. **Discover Unicorn Goods' vast selection of vegan fashion at unicorngoods.com.**

VEGAN MODEL AND SUSTAINABILITY/ ANIMAL-RIGHTS ACTIVIST

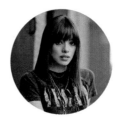

"When my ethics changed, so did my goals and my role in the fashion industry."

She graces the fashion campaigns of ethical brands and uses her influence to speak out against animal abuse, promote veganism, and discuss sustainability in fashion. Rachel Ford is a rare breath of fresh air in the fashion industry:

I became vegan completely out of the blue about two and a half years ago. I came home from work one night, drive-thru McDonald's in hand for a late-night dinner—nothing new. But in what now seems like some kind of divine intervention, my boyfriend and I randomly decided to watch *Food, Inc.* on Netflix. It's not even a vegan film, but that's all it took for me. I was horrified to actually see where my food came from, and what unnecessary cruelty I was supporting. Needless to say, that was the last time I ever ate McDonald's, or any meat for that matter. I chose to

become vegan that night, and it was the easiest and best decision I've ever made.

Veganism is not just a diet, it's a lifestyle. So, when my ethics changed, so did my goals and my role in the fashion industry. While I may not be able to choose all my jobs just yet, there are certain things I just won't do. I'll deny auditions, even paid work, if it directly goes against my beliefs. My job is no longer just about me; it's about furthering the movement. I've decided to turn my career as a model into a platform for activism, as I feel compelled to spread the awareness that transformed my life.

I don't always have the pleasure of choosing the brands I work with. Modeling is my job; it's how I pay the bills. So unfortunately, not all of my clients are ethical brands. Now, I would never work for a leather or fur company, of course—but the abundance of animal products in the industry does make it tough to avoid them sometimes. I would love nothing more than to only work for conscious companies with fellow changemakers who share my values for people, animals, and the planet. However, I am grateful to have met and worked with a few local vegan businesses here in LA. I can't tell you how amazing it feels to combine my personal values and my job.

My best work is when I'm working for a cause I believe in. It ignites this fiery passion within my soul to be the change I wish to see in the world. I've met some fantastic people behind these ethical fashion brands. You can feel the sense of love, compassion, and community in everything they do.

I'm learning to embrace the journey and do my part to inspire and spread cruelty-free culture whenever I can.

From the beginning, Sica Schmitz, founder of Bead & Reel, has been a light in my life. She has given me many opportunities within the ethical fashion industry, introduced me to many like-minded veganistas, and helped me grow along my journey, whether it be sustainable e-commerce for her online boutique or walking in her annual sustainable Fair Trade Fashion Show. She is a modern-day Wonder Woman who I aspire to be like, fighting for social and environmental justice.

Nowadays, I look at my job very differently. While, essentially, I play dress up and take photos—which I love, don't get me wrong—it's not always all fun for me anymore. Before, I mentioned that there are certain factors I cannot control, and that can be tough. For instance, when I have to get my hair and makeup done, it's such a bittersweet feeling. On the one hand I enjoy it, but on the other hand, I'm cringing inside as these toxic, animal-based products are being sprayed on and blended into my skin. Or maybe my only shoe options at work for the day are leather. It's hard having to compromise on issues that completely oppose my personal life and values. But I'm learning that I can only help what I can control. So, I take these opportunities to strike up conversations about my favorite plant-based products, or my vegan leather shoes. Instead of feeling hypocritical about the challenges I face at work, I'm learning to embrace the journey and do my part to inspire and spread cruelty-free culture whenever I can. **Follow Rachel on Instagram at @itsrachelford.**

KOMIE AND MEG VORA

COFOUNDERS OF DELIKATE RAYNE

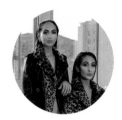

"We felt an area of vacancy when it came to completely cruelty-free and/or eco-friendly pieces."

Sisters Komie and Meg Vora are the creators of vegan apparel brand Delikate Rayne, which caters to an edgier customer with contemporary taste. Since launching their label, the sisters have styled a fashion lookbook for PETA India.

MV: We don't come from a fashion background at all. I have degrees in business and communications, and I was working at a tech startup that specialized in practice management— basically the farthest thing from fashion—before launching the label with Komie.

KV: I received a degree in business and marketing from the Marshall School of Business at USC. Before starting Delikate Rayne, I was a bit closer to a creative field since I was working for an indie jewelry designer who operated from a direct-to-consumer site. My experience there with e-commerce and

online marketing has been beneficial for me with our company.

We wanted to create a new kind of luxury—something that was peaceful and didn't have to sacrifice a life to create a product.

MV: Being born and raised strict vegetarians played a role in the way we viewed many things around us growing up. Fashion ended up being a concept that we would continually revisit and question but couldn't find sufficient answers for when it came to ethics, cruelty-free components, and an aesthetic and style that we felt drawn to. Out of this came our label, and the opportunity to build a completely animal-friendly wardrobe, which has always been one of our major goals.

There have been huge, positive strides toward permanently removing fur from fashion. Many of the larger, mainstream luxury houses have pledged to go fur-free, which marked a monumental moment for those, like us,

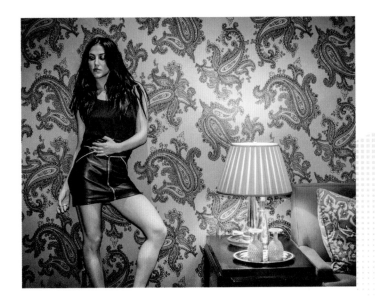

who have been tirelessly fighting for it. It created a chain reaction, and now, more and more major fashion brands are joining in. There's still work to be done when it comes to leather, silk, and wool, etc., but the removal of fur has been a much-needed step in the right direction.

Another win in our favor is the banning of the sale of fur in San Francisco and Los Angeles. With this step, LA became the largest city in the United States to ban the sale of new fur, and we're proud to say that we live here and witnessed the forward momentum firsthand. In addition, many wonderful, innovative, cruelty-free textiles have entered the market, especially for leather (including fabric made out of mushrooms, apple peels, pineapple leaves, kombucha tea, and more) and silk (made out of banana stalks, synthetic spider silk, and so on).

Being a vegan designer is an ongoing battle. We must change the preconceived notions of what luxury is and how animal-friendly clothing is just as good in quality, style, look, and feel as its non-vegan counterparts.

What are your own favorite pieces from your collection?
MV: Right now, it would be our mock-croc vegan leather skirt in red, the silky satin tie top in black, and our "Peace begins with compassion" T-shirt cut into a crop top.

KV: Currently, it's our front-zip vegan leather miniskirt in navy blue, the satin-trim shorts in black, and our limited-edition leopard faux-fur moto jacket.
See the collection at delikaterayne.com.

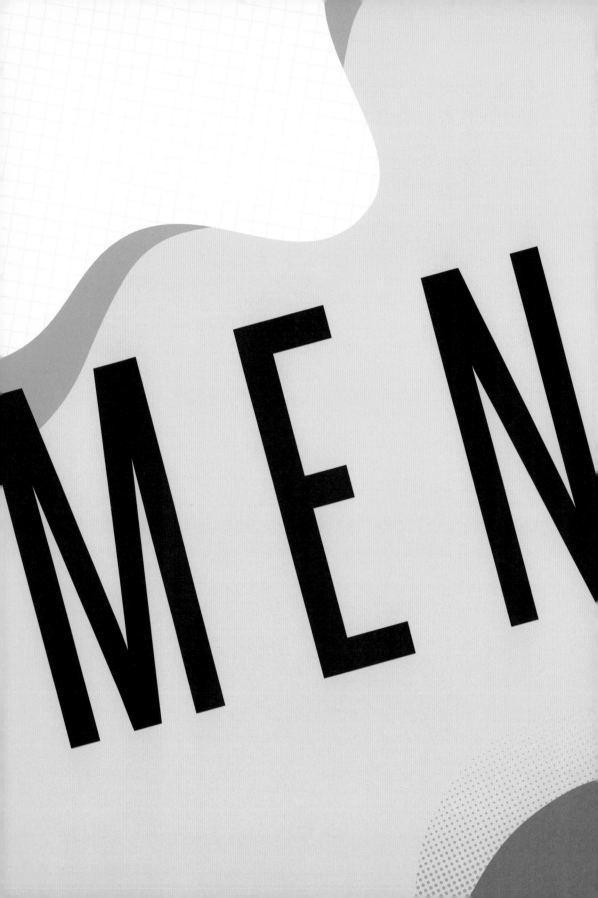

FOR THE GENTLE MAN

Because kind
fashion is hardly
a female-only
pursuit.

Despite the simple fact that most humans in our society wear clothes every day, fashion has, for a long time, been seen as a women's domain.

We're the ones who are expected to be interested in it and excited by it, even though we're certainly not the only sex to have to decide what to wear every morning. Most fashion magazines are aimed at women, as is any television show that focuses on style, and a large percentage of fashion-brand communication. Our society also views it as a given that women enjoy shopping (although many don't) and that men are bored by it (many aren't).

This discrepancy is also reflected in the retail offerings. For many reasons, men's fashion still has some catching up to do. As my husband has remarked on several occasions, "Each fashion store is overflowing with women's clothing—with a boring, black-and-gray corner hidden away somewhere, with an arrow labelled 'men' pointing to it, making it even more difficult for men to enjoy shopping." Many shops bury their menswear in the basement or the remote second or third floor, letting women's fashion take center stage.

But the stylish men of the world are rebelling against female domination in fashion. These days, men's style is stepping out of the shadow of women's fashion and finding its own feet. Being interested in fashion and having a distinct style as a dude is more accepted than

VEGAN STYLE

ever. Stylish men no longer simply suit up—they now experiment with colors, patterns, and textiles almost as much as their female counterparts. Male fashion bloggers are building audiences to rival those of the ladies', and male fashion magazines are considered almost as influential as female-led ones. Men's fashion weeks are attracting crowds, and male celebrities are more creative than ever with their style—forget wearing the same old black suit to every awards show: that's so 2009. Today's male trendsetters rock runway looks taken straight from the catwalks in New York, London, Milan, and Paris—and they look great doing it.

It's sort of the same thing with veganism and vegetarianism. At one point, it was the domain of cool celebrities like Tobey Maguire and Jared Leto, athletes like David Haye and Nate Diaz, outspoken activists like James Aspey and rock stars Rise Against and Blink-182, and Daniel Johns of Australian band Silverchair. Being a vegetarian or vegan was seen as something that women did—living compassionately is, after all, a way of showing that you care. And, while straight women all over the planet know that the sexiest thing a man can do is show emotion, the word hadn't quite spread among the menfolk. Until now. All of a sudden, being vegan is not only accepted in male circles, it's viewed as a cool, alternative, and rebellious move.

It is therefore hardly surprising that vegan style is branching out into men's territory too—there is endless scope for turning the traditionally wool- and leather-rich menswear realm vegan-friendly, and there is so much ground to cover with innovative, sustainable materials. In this chapter, we'll take a look at what men's vegan fashion looks like now, and how it is likely to evolve.

MEN

VEGAN STYLE ESSENTIALS

It's never been easier—or more exciting—to create a capsule wardrobe as a man who wishes to dress consciously. By looking outside the mall and the big-name retailers, and taking another look at smaller, more up-and-coming brands that create ethical fashion for men, you will soon find that you're the best-dressed one among your friends— and you'll be doing it all without harming animals. For your new and improved wardrobe, look no further than these pioneering brands.

best for

SUITS

▽

Brave GentleMan

Sharp and well cut, the styles offered by Joshua Katcher (see page 184) are every bit as dapper as their woolly counterparts, if not more so. "Future wool," as Joshua calls the material his suits are cut from, is 100 percent animal-free. It's crafted from recycled polyester and cotton blends, color-separated for a dye-free process.

best for

SHOES

▽

Bourgeois Boheme

Bourgeois Boheme is a shoe brand for all your needs, be it sneakers or more formal styles. The London-based brand's men's range is a cut above the rest: from dapper Derby designs to Chelsea boots and sneakers in Piñatex, the vegan leather material made from waste pineapple fibers. These are styles that don't scream "vegan shoes," but quietly whisper: "I'm a man who knows how to dress."

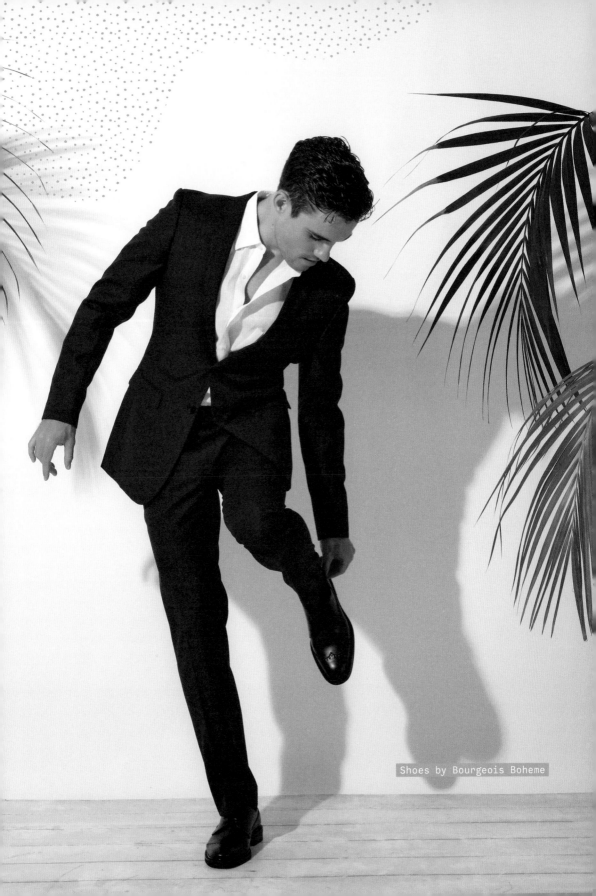

Shoes by Bourgeois Boheme

JEANS

Monkee Genes

This PETA-approved vegan brand is
not only kind to animals but is also
produced with care for humans and
the planet; their organic range is free
from pesticides and toxic chemicals.
Choose from their vast array of
conscious designs for a pair of long-
lasting jeans that will stay in your
wardrobe for ages.

best for

T-SHIRTS

Everlane

San Francisco–based sustainable
fashion brand Everlane is known for
being dedicated to transparency—in
fact, when you shop on their
website, you can see exactly where
in the world your purchase was
created, down to the very factory
that crafted the cotton for your
Oxford button-down shirt. The
designs are clean, classic, and
perfect for matching with everything
from formalwear to weekend attire.

best for

BRIEFCASES

Matt & Nat

The perfect addition to a sleek
workwear suit, Matt & Nat's
eco-friendly selection of
briefcases is a winner when it
comes to both quality and style.
Offering a variety of elegant,
muted shades, Matt & Nat is your
go-to brand for accessorizing
with effortless class.

KNITWEAR

Bleed

There are things we like about the cold-weather
months, and things we dislike. Thick, heavy
knitwear is up there with hot chocolates on the
relatively short "good things about chilly weather"
list. Good news: PETA-approved vegan brand Bleed
creates organic and fairly produced knitwear
inspired by sportswear and mountain life in that
relaxed, soft fit we all love to snuggle up in over
the winter. Tip: wear these designs with your
Monkee Genes (see opposite).

best for

LONG-SLEEVED SHIRTS

Thought

This menswear company actually evolved to include
womenswear, not the other way around, and it offers
everyday essentials free from harmful pesticides and
toxic chemicals. They're not entirely vegan—some wool
does creep in—but you can find plenty of cotton,
bamboo, and hemp fabrics as well as the odd piece in
Tencel and Modal. Whether you're a fan of stripes or
block colors, V-necks or round ones, chances are that
elusive weekend top is waiting for you here.

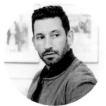

JOSHUA KATCHER

FOUNDER OF BRAVE GENTLEMAN,
ADJUNCT PROFESSOR AT PARSONS
SCHOOL OF DESIGN, AND BLOGGER
AT THE DISCERNING BRUTE

"I went into fashion as an activist."

As an adjunct professor at the Parsons School of Design, Joshua Katcher is a fashion insider. But he's also as rare as a vegan in the fashion industry. Having founded leading men's vegan fashion website The Discerning Brute, Joshua was one of the first voices to speak about ethical fashion for men. He is also the founder of vegan fashion brand Brave GentleMan, whose shoes have been worn by Jared Leto.

I went into fashion as an activist. I realized that fashion was a powerful tool that not only shaped identity but was a global industrial complex reshaping animals and the environment on an enormous scale. As an activist, I was always looking for the most effective way to reach people—not just to shake my finger at them but to reach them in a way that sidesteps the defensive reaction that so many people have to information that challenges their worldview. Fashion, I thought, is one of those things that is seductive, aspirational, and immediate. Vegan fashion is an argument and solution that is aesthetically rational. In other words, the beauty of a fashion object can reflect the beauty of how it's made.

For a long time, veganism was viewed as not only a giving-up of pleasure but also as an antithesis of patriarchal power. Compassion and empathy are often seen as feminine qualities in our culture, and are therefore associated with weaknesses. I used The Discerning Brute to subvert notions of mainstream masculinity and to package compassion for animals for a GQ-type audience. There were skeptics and critics, of course, but mostly there were people who were really happy that I was confronting masculinity and speaking to men about living not just "the good life" but "the better life." There was a sense of relief and validation.

Now, many vegan products are seen as just as good if not better than those that use animal materials. It's been exciting to see this transformation happen, and to have played a part in it. Vegan fashion is a methodology, not an aesthetic. And now we're on the cusp of the most exciting material innovations since the industrial revolution. Synthetic biology is about to change the way we make everything, and soon, raising animals for their skins and hair will be obsolete.

We're on the cusp of the most exciting material innovations since the industrial revolution.

There is some prejudice that vegan fashion is a limitation, a sacrifice of pleasure and beauty, and something "fake." This is partly our own fault for continuing to use words like "faux," "fake," "alternative," etc., when we should be using words like "superior," "future," and "beyond." Leather is not inherently better than vegan leather. In fact, certain vegan leather outperforms animal skin in durability and customizability. This is a marketing problem that some of us are working hard on.

The biggest challenge for men's ethical fashion today is identity. What it means to be a man is very tied up in notions of brutishness. Aspiring toward power also crosses over into women's fashion with items like fur coats or exotic-skin heels. For example, the rarer an animal or the crueller a process, the more valuable a material is perceived to be because having it is a demonstration of access, of economic power, and of a willingness to be ruthless. This can be traced back to European royalty of the Middle Ages and their ermine capes, for example, that required hundreds of animals that lived in a far-off place and who were difficult to hunt to be turned into a singular garment. It's all about power and being perceived as powerful. Until vegan fashion can become a symbol of power, it's going to be a tough sell in the context of our current culture, whose preferences lean more toward sports cars with leather seats, snorting rhino horn powder, and owning a crocodile watchband or a vicuña sweater.

GROOMING
for the compassionate man

As male grooming trends continue to grow—boy beautification is now a booming, multibillion-dollar industry worldwide—vegan-friendly personal-care brands are amplifying their offerings for men by branching out into beard products, face washes, and moisturizers with a masculine touch. If you're a compassionate dude, or looking for a gift for one, here are a few labels to note.

Bulldog

This "man's best friend" British brand proudly proclaims its preference for natural ingredients and, in fact, came about when founder Simon Duffy spotted a gap in the market for male personal-care products made from natural ingredients. This led him to create Bulldog's range of nontoxic, paraben-free products that are certified by both Cruelty Free International and the Vegetarian Society. Bulldog offers gift sets that make perfect presents for compassionate men—maybe try gifting one to a man who doesn't know much about vegan grooming and watch him fall in love with it.

D + T Organic Beard Care

Australian David Rafter was tired of the lack of vegan-friendly grooming options for men—so he created this sophisticated, minimalist beard-care brand featuring only organic and cruelty-free ingredients.

●

LUSH

It's the go-to brand for natural cosmetics—their signature bath bombs are a huge hit with, well, everyone who's got access to a bathtub. And the next time you pay a visit to one of their sweet-smelling beauty shops, take note of the men's product selection: these days, the LUSH selection for dudes is (almost) as impressive as the one for the ladies. From ocean-salt face cleansers to cocoa-butter moisturizers and face masks (which are marketed with a message no man can argue with: "If Batman wore a mask, why can't you?"), this is the one brand that will solve all your vegan-man grooming issues.

●

Brooklyn Grooming

This stateside men's face- and body-care label offers organic, vegan, and cruelty-free facial products, beard balms and oils, and beard tools. Its hipster packaging will add flair to the vegan man's bathroom cabinet, and the nontoxic ingredients are good for your health as well as your look.

●

The Body Shop

Our beloved Body Shop has a pretty much fifty-fifty split of male and female products these days. Despite being a longtime leader of the fight against animal testing, The Body Shop does not sell a completely vegan range; however, many of the products are vegan-friendly, and all are cruelty-free. Products to try: the entire Activist line for men is vegan, and so is the White Musk for Men series, featuring aftershave, deodorant, and eau de toilette.

FOUNDER OF WILL'S VEGAN SHOES

"I wanted to make shoes people fell in love with."

Entrepreneur Will Green does not look like your typical vegan. In fact, this dapper Londoner embodies the definition of a stylish modern man—but, when he decided to follow his passion and launch a shoe brand, he knew exactly what kind of accessories he wanted to offer: affordable, fashion-forward styles that didn't contain any animal products, and that were also kind to the planet. This is how Will's Vegan Shoes was born. Aside from their range of shoes for men, women, and children, the brand also offers bags, backpacks, belts, and more.

Needless to say, all Will's designs are vegan, but aside from this, they are also ethically produced in Portugal, where workers' conditions are safe and salaries are fair. Those things matter to Will as much as keeping it animal-friendly, which makes his collection an all-around winner for those looking to shop kind fashion. Here's what he had to say:

I have always wanted to make a difference with my life. I was brought up in a free-thinking vegetarian family, have always loved the idea of having my own shop, and held a passion for shoes. Everything came together while working for another vegan shoe company. People kept telling me how hard it was to buy ethical and fashionable, affordable shoes. I knew what the steps were to make my own vegan shoes, so took the leap and started Will's Vegan Shoes in spring 2013. I wanted to make shoes that people fell in love with; the kind of shoes you would want to wear even if they didn't go with your outfit.

I travel around Europe searching for the best vegan materials, such as

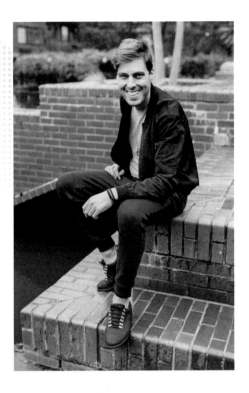

beautiful Italian microfiber uppers and linings. I've noticed the first thing some people do when they pick up a pair of Will's is smell them to check for leather, because they cannot believe they're vegan.

I make my shoes in top factories in Portugal, where people work in decent, safe conditions and are paid a fair wage. I place animal and human rights on the same level; I don't see the point of protecting one life and putting another in danger. I embedded my ethics in my company, which is why my shoes are and always will be vegan and ethically made.

My inspiration comes from living in London and seeing what people are wearing. My shoes are a kind of reaction to that experience. I rarely have time to check what the shops are selling, what is shown at the exhibits, or what is supposed to be "big" next season.

Cruelty-free fashion could and should go all the way. Whether this happens, I think, is up to us. I don't think that we realize the power we have. If we all took responsibility for our personal actions, we could change everything. Do you think the sweatshop industry would last one week if everyone stopped buying £5 ($9) shoes tomorrow? Would chemicals be put into our food chain if we all chose to buy organic? Would animals be murdered if we all stopped eating meat? Look at the biggest positive changes in the world in the last two hundred years—they all began with the individual.

My dream is to bridge the gap between everyday people and ethically produced vegan shoes.

FAQS

Everything you wanted to know about vegan fashion but had no idea who to ask.

THE ESSENTIAL KNOW-HOW FOR A VEGAN LIFE

Transitioning to a cruelty-free life—and wardrobe—will inevitably elicit questions.

I remember when I first realized that I had to check all my winter knitwear for wool from now on—and having lived in cold, Northern European countries for most of my life, that was a lot of knitwear. To be honest, it was kind of a relief; wool knits tend to sting. Another surprise came when I realized that I had to check my shoes for three different components—the sole, the upper, and the insole. Leather can lurk in any of these three components, and it's not always clear whether all parts of the shoe are vegan or not.

Like any other lifestyle change, overhauling your wardrobe can be daunting and is best taken one step at a time. Finding new places to shop (I basically had to abandon all the places I'd been shopping for beauty, for example, and find new ones) and exploring new brands are the exciting bits of transitioning your wardrobe. But, of course, a lifestyle change like this is gradual and, as you go along, you might find yourself wondering about everything from Chinese animal testing laws to the best ways to clean faux fur. No worries—I've done my best to be your guide to the exciting (and sometimes a bit confusing) world of cruelty-free living.

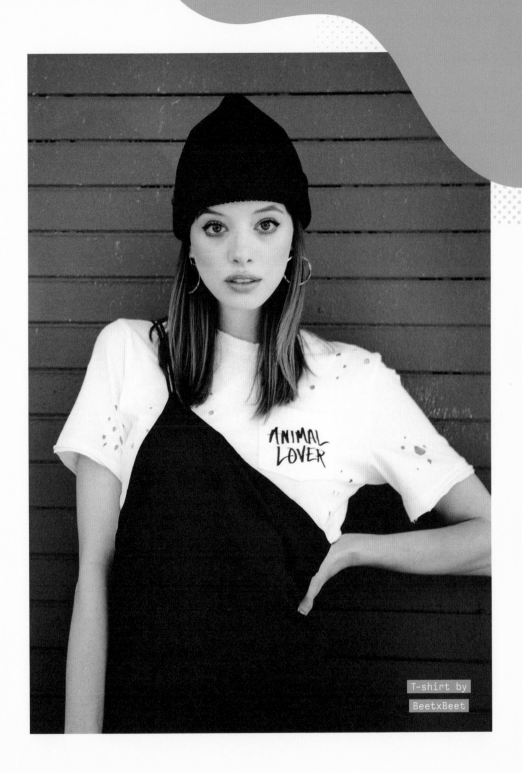

T-shirt by
BeetxBeet

193

FAQS

SHOPPING

Q WHERE CAN I SHOP THE BEST VEGAN FASHION ONLINE?

A Where do I start? When I was transitioning to a vegan wardrobe, it was slim pickings. But these days, shopping for vegan fashion is a whole new world. If you want to support ethical style and small, often female-owned businesses, check out these multibrand retailers:

Bead & Reel

A 100 percent vegan, ethical, and sustainable online fashion boutique run by former Hollywood costume designer Sica Schmitz (for more on Sica, see page 158). Sica uses a range of criteria to choose the products that feature on Bead & Reel: ethical, vegan, locally produced, fair trade, and female-founded are a few areas that the brand supports.
Brands include: BHAVA, Nae, Passion Lillie (beadandreel.com)

Nois New York

A contemporary, curated collection of vegan apparel and accessories. Nois is an ethical retailer bringing modern, sustainable style to the New York fashion insiders—and its clean, minimalist aesthetic has won fans all over the globe.
Brands include: Matt & Nat, Kowtow, Susi Studio

T H R I V E

A Swedish online boutique dedicated to sustainable, ethical, and vegan fashion. T H R I V E features an impressive selection of both menswear and womenswear, including an extensive range of denim—all PETA-approved vegan. Inject some Scandi style into your look with the cruelty-free selection from this cool and compassionate shop.
Brands include: HoodLamb, Bourgeois Boheme, Ethletic (thrivestore.se)

Modavanti

This is not a 100 percent vegan shop, but if you want to shop vegan fashion, it's still a great place to click onto. Meaning "fashion forward" in Italian, this online retailer specializes in eco-friendly fashion made with care for the planet and respect for workers. Fair trade, recycled, and locally produced are some of the criteria for the fashions sold by Modavanti. Brands include: Angela Roi, People Tree, Will's Vegan Shoes (modavanti.com)

Unicorn Goods

The world's biggest online catalog for vegan fashion. The website collates cruelty-free fashion for men and women in a superstore that will bring you plenty of inspiration—if you had any doubts about how much fun (and not at all limiting) cruelty-free shopping could be, Unicorn Goods is your reminder. Brands include: VAUTE, Mechaly, Reformation (unicorngoods.com)

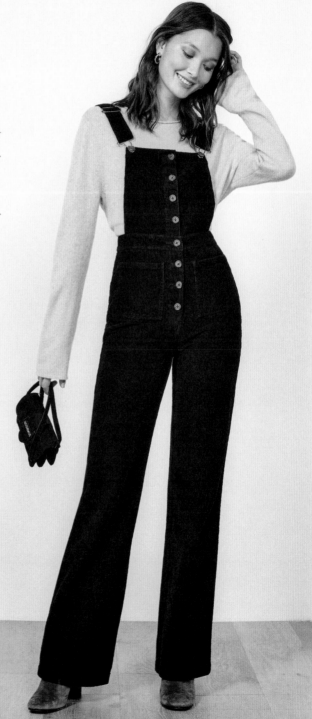

Dungarees by Reformation

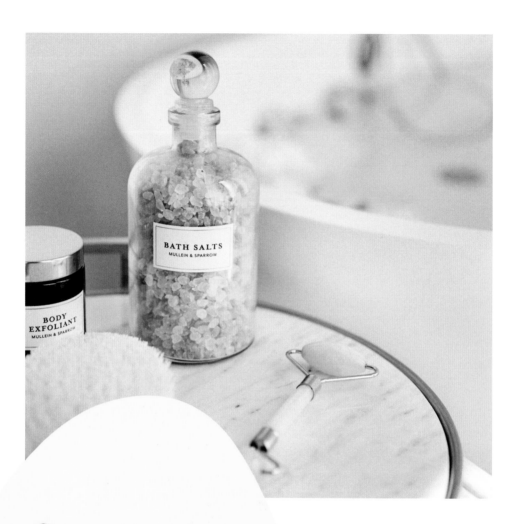

Q WHAT ABOUT VEGAN BEAUTY?

A Warning: online shops that carry vegan beauty products are addictive. You will be sucked into an endless black hole of buying products that you had no idea you needed. There are vegan versions of absolutely every product you can possibly imagine—and often they smell better than the non-vegan versions you were familiar with.

Flora & Fauna

An Australian beauty and health boutique that goes above and beyond in their ethical aim. The brand's goal is to be a zero-waste business by using plastic-free products and packaging, and by making sure that all packaging and containers have a recyclable option. All the products are 100 percent vegan, and the brand has partnerships with charities such as Sea Shepherd as well as animal shelters.
(floraandfauna.com.au)

Petit Vour

A US-based monthly subscription box offering a selection of vegan beauty products on a monthly basis (see page 124). Once you click on the luxuriously beautiful website, you get to create your beauty profile with characteristics that fit your skin, body, and hair, so that your monthly curated box suits your needs. You can also shop vegan fashion and lifestyle items and earn PV points to spend in the shop by reviewing boxes.
(petitvour.com)

LoveLula

A British-based marketplace for organic cosmetics, refusing any use of toxic substances like parabens or SLS, and any use of animal testing. Many of the products offered by LoveLula are also vegan, and clearly marked on the site as such. Some are certified by the Soil Association (meaning that over 71 percent of the ingredients are organic) and Ecocert (meaning that 95 percent of the ingredients are natural and vegetable, and at least 10 percent are organic).
(lovelula.com)

Credo Beauty

Not 100 percent vegan, but has a very good vegan selection. Focusing on "clean beauty," Credo offers nontoxic and cruelty-free products with a holistic vision. Animal-derived ingredients are at the top of their "dirty" ingredients list, but beeswax and lanolin might pop up in some of their items, so read the label.
(credobeauty.com)

Q WHY ARE ETHICAL BRANDS SO EXPENSIVE?

A This has been on my mind so many times—transitioning to ethically produced fashion was a real process for me, and it took (and is taking) a long time because sustainable fashion is considerably more expensive than so-called fast fashion. The difference in price is owed to the fact that the garment's production circumstances and processes are simply better than those of cheaper fashion. Workers are paid decent salaries and work in respectable conditions. The material is processed using practices that tread more lightly on our planet. All of this amounts to a higher price tag on the finished item, but it's worth it.

Djuna Da Silva, founder of New York-based sustainable fashion label Djuna Shay, says:

"If I did the things that a lot of fast-fashion companies do, like make the choice to move production overseas, not investigate labor, use cheaper materials, and not investigate my supply chain, I would have a much more profitable business with much larger margins. However, as someone who knows that there is no planet B, I know that's not an option."

If, like me, you'd love to pay more for the commitment it takes to help make fashion kinder to animals and our planet but just don't have the means, there are ways to be an ethical consumer without breaking the bank.

Have a swap party.
Invite your friends over with instructions to bring clothes they no longer wear, get some wine, and rummage through each other's pre-loved garments. Chances are, one's trash will be another's treasure.

Re-Love what you already have.
Rediscover what's already in your wardrobe by getting creative and composing new outfits with the pieces you already own. That way, you might discover that you actually wish to keep some of the garments you were intent on getting rid of, leading to less shopping and less waste.

How to dress ethically on a budget

Check out your local thrift store.
Buying secondhand is one of the best ways to stay cruelty-free on a budget. It's a very exciting way to shop, too; you never know what gems you will find.

Shop secondhand.
Pre-loved clothing is a great way to renew your style without putting any new strain on the planet's resources—and it will save you some money, too. Check out apps like Depop (a favorite of many style bloggers), eBay, HEWI (Hardly Ever Worn It), and ASOS Marketplace for garments that someone else decided to part ways with but that might find a new home in your wardrobe.

FAQS

MATERIALS

Q BUT ISN'T FAUX FUR BAD FOR THE ENVIRONMENT?

A Wearing any kind of fur, real or fake, is not ideal from an environmentalist point of view; faux fur is often made from petroleum-based plastics that don't biodegrade. So, if you want to be as eco-friendly as possible, there's always the option of not wearing any fur at all and going for a sustainably produced wool-free winter coat instead. That said, studies show that faux fur is considerably less harmful to the environment than real fur: a Dutch study from 2013 showed that "a natural mink fur product will always have a larger environmental impact than faux fur"—five times more impact on the environment than the second-highest scoring textile, which is wool. The study determined the impact of fur production in relation to eighteen different environmental issues, such as climate change, soil acidification, ozone pollution, and water and land use, comparing it to other commonly used materials in fashion production. For seventeen of the eighteen issues, fur was found to be much more harmful than textiles.

The environmental impacts of real fur are tied to the fact that any animals used in the trade will produce manure, which can pollute waterways. Pro-fur arguments may include the fact that fur is biodegradable, but that is only because fur, just like leather or any skin, begins the decaying process as soon as it's taken off the animal. In order to keep the fur from "biodegrading" (i.e., rotting), a host of chemicals such as formaldehyde and ethoxylates are used to treat it, making fur potentially toxic and an environmental hazard.

More good news for eco-friendly lovers of faux fur: French faux-fur artisans Ecopel are introducing a faux-fur fabric made from recycled plastic bottles. Thanks to their new collection system at their mills in Asia, the brand is now able to source post-consumer bottles that will be given new life as faux-fur coats.

Q ISN'T LEATHER THE ENVIRONMENTALLY FRIENDLY CHOICE?

A Leather, a global killer that claims the lives of over one billion animals per year, is also an eco-villain. The tanning process involves chemicals such as hexavalent chromium (yep, the kind Julia Roberts waged war against in *Erin Brockovich*), causing 90 percent of tannery workers in Bangladesh—where much of the world's leather is produced—to die before the age of fifty. Many of these workers are children. The Blacksmith Institute, a nonprofit group that works to reduce pollution in developing nations, included tanneries on its 2012 list of the world's top ten toxic industries. The 2017 Pulse of Fashion Industry report showed that leather is the most environmentally harmful material among all surveyed for cradle-to-gate impact (meaning from the obtaining of the raw materials until the product reaches the consumer). Brands who use vegetable-tanned leather make a tiny difference, but the 2017 Kering Environmental Profit & Loss Report found that 93 percent of all the environmental damage of leather occurs before we even get to the tannery stage, due to the damage of raising animals for leather.

Because leather production is so unsafe, it's hardly even practiced in the US and Europe, and operations are moving overseas—risking the health of people in developing countries so that consumers in the West can enjoy wearing leather shoes and carrying leather bags.

And consider this: leather is almost impossible to trace. Despite the tag saying "made in France/Italy," this only refers to where the garment was assembled. There is no way to know where, and which animal, the actual leather came from. Since so much fur and leather comes from China, where a thriving dog and cat leather industry exists (see page 61), there is no way of knowing exactly what you're wearing—that nonspecified "genuine leather" might, in fact, come from a dog or a cat.

Q DOESN'T IT MAKE SENSE TO USE THE WHOLE ANIMAL IF LEATHER COMES FROM THE MEAT INDUSTRY?

A If you eat meat, then of course buying and wearing leather takes on another meaning than it would for a vegan. But even so, cutting out one thing is better than doing nothing. Baby steps are the way forward. But is leather really a meat by-product? It can be, but the whole truth isn't that simple. Cowhides are more expensive than meat, meaning that leather has a value and a market all its own, independent from the meat industry. This value is reflected in the treatment of many cows bred for their leather: if you look at video footage of cows slaughtered in Bangladesh—where so much of today's leather comes from—you will see just how skinny and emaciated the cows are. From a moral point of view, the debate around using a whole animal matters very little when the animal in question has the right to live free from suffering.

What about vintage fur and leather?

I'm torn on this one, and I know that many others are with me. Vintage is better than new. Personally, I wouldn't wear it—but I wouldn't condemn those wearing vintage leather as much as I would those opting for newly produced leather. I know some vegans disagree with me, and I very much respect that—from an environmental standpoint, vintage wins all the way over newly produced. But remember that it doesn't matter when an animal died. Whether it was yesterday or thirty years ago, the skin on your back came from an animal that deserved to live his or her life. Also, the fur you inherited doesn't come with a label saying "I'm vintage."

Q ISN'T WOOL JUST A HAIRCUT FOR THE SHEEP?

A Wool is often seen as the "kind" fabric—it's natural, it's warm, and you don't need to kill the animal to use it. Win-win, right? Wrong. As many undercover investigations have proved, wool production, just like any production where animals are used on a large scale, can't be cruelty-free due to the fact that the animals are treated like commodities, which means that their well-being is never considered as much as the money-making. Workers in the wool industry are often paid by volume, not by the hour, so they need to work quickly and obtain as much wool as possible. This is as far from a haircut as you can imagine (unless your hairdresser is some kind of sadist). Sheep are often nicked and cut in the process and left with bleeding wounds—some of which are sometimes sewn up with a thread and needle with no pain relief (I'm wincing as I type this). They suffer from infections and are often denied basic veterinary care. And that's all before even mentioning flystrike and mulesing (see page 31). Plus, it's not entirely correct to claim that wool is produced without killing animals. When a sheep's abused body is considered "spent" and can no longer produce wool, it is, of course, sent to the slaughterhouse.

Why not silk?

Silk is known for being supremely soft and truly high in quality. When you're shopping for a big-ticket dress, silk usually takes center stage. But where does silk actually come from, and why do vegans stay away from it?

The fabric of silk comes from the thread woven by silkworms to make their cocoons. In order to obtain silk, the cocoons are boiled, with the silkworms inside being boiled alive. It takes the lives of 30,000 silk worms to create just one silk blouse. If we want to avoid hurting cows, fish, pigs, fur-bearing animals, and/or worms, we should consider that a worm can suffer just as much as any other animal.

Informing
yourself is
key to making
conscious
consumer
choices.

What are some ethical vegan materials?

How much time have you got? The possibilities are endless, and every day new progress is made. A few examples (read more about this on page 221–22) include:

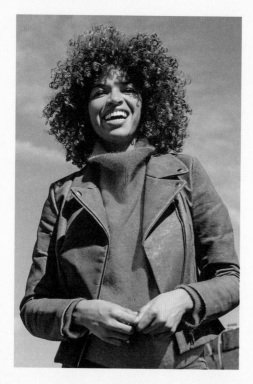

Ovide's sustainable vegan biker jackets are made from cork.
~~~

PIÑATEX
A leather alternative made from waste pineapple-leaf fibers (see page 222).

MUSKIN
A leather made from mushrooms (see page 221).

KOMBUCHA
A leather made from kombucha tea (see page 222).

CORK
One of the eco-friendliest leather replacements out there (see page 221).

TENCEL
A silk and wool replacement made from the cellulose found in eucalyptus trees.

HEMP
A natural material that can be used to replace wool.

LINEN
An airy and breezy natural fabric to replace silk.

COTTON
Just make sure it's organic (see page 44).

ETHICS

Q WHY DO SOME BEAUTY BRANDS SAY THEY ARE CRUELTY-FREE BUT THEN SELL IN CHINA?

A What cruelty-free actually means is a tricky area: in 2013, a ban on cosmetics testing was introduced in Europe, causing animal lovers everywhere to rejoice—and numerous brands to proclaim that they "didn't test on animals." But even if a company's product or ingredients have not been tested in the EU, you have no way of knowing if the product is cruelty-free until you get the answer to a very important question: Does the brand in question sell their products in China?

China is a huge and very important market to the cosmetics industry, and it's not a market that many brands are willing to ignore. However, Chinese regulations require that any cosmetics products sold in the territory be subjected to a variety of tests, including tests on animals. So, if the brand you're buying from sells their products in China, they will certainly have been tested on animals. This is why the cruelty-free lists that we covered on pages 120–21 do not include brands that sell cosmetics there, and the entities we discussed in that chapter (see page 106) are all working with Chinese authorities to consider alternatives to animal testing.

The wording to look out for if you aren't sure about a brand is this: "We never test our products or ingredients on animals unless required by law." These last words are what effectively makes a company non-cruelty free, as it refers to selling in China.

Also, keep in mind that this only applies to products sold in China—not necessarily those manufactured there. I was terrified once upon seeing the words "Made in China" on my Barry M mascara, only to learn that the brand doesn't actually sell their cosmetics there, and so has the option not to test on animals.

Q WHAT ABOUT CHEAP BRANDS WITH MANY VEGAN OPTIONS, BUT EVEN MORE HUMAN-RIGHTS VIOLATIONS?

A It's a very tricky balance, and hard to always get right, so don't beat yourself up if you find out you slipped up somewhere. You live and you learn. So-called fast fashion brands often get slapped with all the criticism for environmental harm and human-rights issues, but we tend to let "luxury" fashion off the hook, which isn't entirely correct. Operating from a point of view that volumes are smaller is only half the truth—I've seen luxury consumers invade Milan at certain times of the year to shop their own weight in Gucci and Louis Vuitton. Many of these high spenders will never wear their new purchases beyond the current season. In 2016, Fashion Revolution, in partnership with Ethical Consumer, launched the Fashion Transparency Index, a report that ranks clothing brands on their transparency. It uses a ratings methodology that benchmarks companies against current and basic best practice in supply chain transparency in five key areas: policy and commitment; tracking and traceability; audits and remediation; engagement and collaboration; and governance. The results were divided into "low rating," meaning little to no evidence that the company has more than a Code of Conduct in place—companies with this rating are making little effort toward being transparent about their supply chain practices; "low-middle/high-middle rating"; and "top rating," where companies are making significant efforts in the given areas and have made some or most of this information publicly available.

All luxury companies on the global top ten of the largest fashion companies, including LVMH, Hermés, and Chanel, were evaluated with "low rating," along with fast-fashion companies like Forever 21. Among the "top rating" appear Zara and H&M. Nike had "high-middle rating." The most valuable and the highest-digit sales companies are also the most lax.

This does in no way mean that fast fashion is innocent. Far from it. Its huge volumes and constant influx of new "collections" (sometimes on a weekly basis) mean that despite being vegan-friendly, shopping with these companies has implications of other kinds, such as human-rights violations, sometimes connections to slavery, and heavy pollution of the environment, which of course also affects animals. Watch the documentary *The True Cost* to find out more about how overconsumption is killing the planet.

In their defense, many of these brands are trying their hand at sustainable collections—H&M Conscious being the first, and Zara Join Life and Mango Committed following. But to be completely certain that you are, in fact, shopping ethically, stick to smaller brands with a higher level of traceability.

CARE

Q HOW DO YOU CARE FOR FAUX LEATHER?

A Caring for faux leather is not that different to caring for the real deal, and with the right care, your faux garments should last you a while. Use a leather cleaner to remove stains, always using a mild detergent afterward and wipe off with a soft, nonabrasive cloth.

Direct sunlight can cause faux leather to crack, and my best tip is to use Vaseline as a "sunscreen" for your faux products. I've seen this work like a charm on my own bags and jackets—it keeps them soft and helps to protect the material from drying out.

Don't ever use bleach on faux leather; it's one of the most drying substances out there, and you will almost certainly harm your garment.

Q HOW DO YOU CLEAN FAUX FUR?

A Good news: you can actually toss your faux fur in the washing machine. Turn it inside out to prevent pilling and tumble-dry with no heat. Of course, if the label on your faux-fur coat or jacket says "dry-clean only," don't throw it in the wash. Respect the label. For me, personally, I usually check that pretty much nothing I buy has that label; I just can't be bothered to take it to the dry cleaners.

Q HOW DO YOU FIX FAUX LEATHER IF IT BREAKS?

A If your faux-leather jacket starts peeling and cracking, try a vinyl and leather repair kit. When my jacket cracked, my husband fixed it with a repair remedy meant for real leather called Magic Mender.

Q HOW DO YOU WASH WOOL-FREE KNITS?

A I wash everything cold, as it's eco-friendlier (most of the greenhouse gas emissions involved in laundry come from warming the water that we use to wash our clothes), but in my own experience there are other benefits to washing with cold water too. Your fake wools, which will often be cotton blended with a synthetic material, will be happy with your chilly choice—they'll stay pill-free and smooth for ages.

Q BEST TIPS TO MAKE INEXPENSIVE SHOES LAST LONGER?

A Bought an inexpensive pair of vegan shoes and want to get as much use out of them as you can? Been there, my friend. As much as we'd all like to be able to afford Stella McCartney Elyse platforms, we often must give in to our wallets. To get more wear out of your purchases, here are a few tips that will make your shoes look like a million bucks on a dime:

GET REINFORCEMENT

Get the toes, heels, and outsoles reinforced. That way, you can protect the sole and especially the heel of the shoe much better. Most heels on cheap shoes are made from plastic, and if you wear down the plastic too quickly, they're harder to replace.

DON'T OVERWEAR

Rotation, rotation, rotation. Wearing the same shoes constantly is the best way to wear them out. Make sure you give your pair a few days' breather before re-wearing.

CLEAN REGULARLY

Get your cleaning routine down. Faux leather is much easier to clean than real leather— use diluted dish detergent or hand soap and wipe with a cloth. Easy, and no need for fancy cleansers.

FAQS

THE VEG

AN-OVER

VEGANIZE YOUR LIFE

How to easily transition to a cruelty-free lifestyle.

When you make the decision to switch to a vegan lifestyle,

the first steps you take are likely to be all about what you eat (and what never to let into your fridge again). Overhauling your diet seems like a big step, but, once it's done, you're often amazed at how easy it was. And then come the thoughts of the next step: How do you go about making your entire life cruelty-free? And, as clothes are such a constant part of our lives, a vegan wardrobe is often the next thing on the list.

Creating a cruelty-free wardrobe doesn't have to mean throwing out every leather jacket and wool sweater you own right away—although if you want to donate or sell your non-vegan clothes and replace them immediately, by all means, go ahead. For most of us, veganizing our wardrobe means gradually replacing items as they wear out to avoid excess waste and spending a fortune all at once. So, don't beat yourself up if you're still wearing your old wool sweater. Just make sure that next time you buy a sweater, it's vegan. It's normal for change to take time.

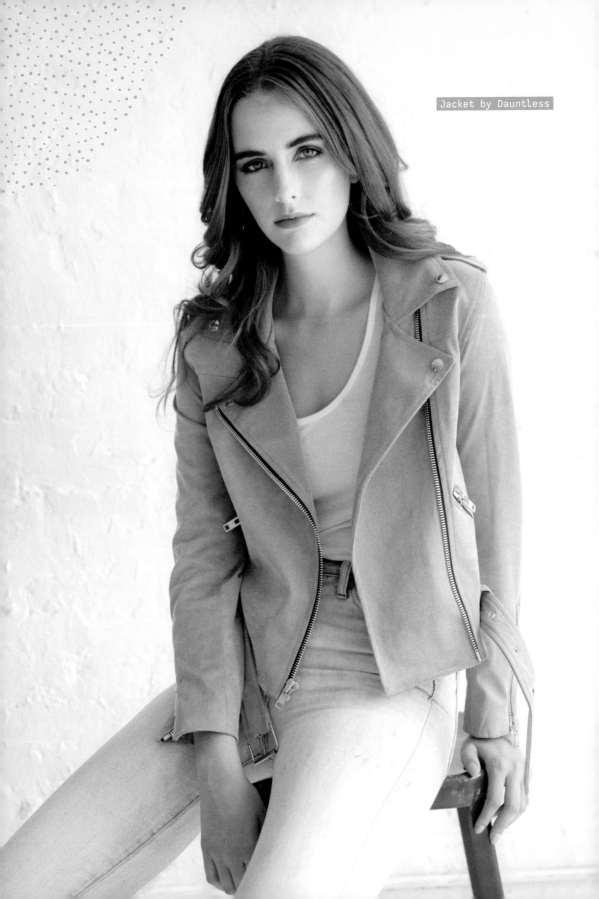

A NOTE ON WASTE

Whatever you do, don't throw out your clothes, no matter how shocked and disgusted you may be upon discovering the truth behind the animal-skins industry. I have sometimes come across stories of people who handled their reaction to the horrors of the skins trade by hauling their entire wardrobe to the dumpster. "I was so horrified," these stories say. "I just couldn't keep these items in my wardrobe, and I felt so relieved once I was rid of them." What these people forget is that throwing away clothing is incredibly harmful to the environment: those leather jackets and woolly knits will only end up in a landfill, which releases toxic greenhouse gases such as carbon dioxide and methane into the atmosphere. Clothing waste is a big environmental hazard, as tons of clothing get thrown away each year. Chucking those clothes, unless there's something irreparably wrong with them (stains that can't be removed, holes, and so on), is wasteful and would truly mean that the animal died for nothing. There are many better ways to transition to a vegan wardrobe that don't involve waste and environmental destruction.

WHAT TO DO WITH THE NON-VEGAN ITEMS YOU CURRENTLY OWN

Your options are to donate, sell, give away, or keep. What you choose to do depends largely on the item, its condition, and its sentimental value to you. If that leather bag you got as a graduation gift from your parents is too close to your heart to sell, but carrying it makes you feel oddly self-conscious and jars with your vegan values, store it as a treasured keepsake in your wardrobe, perhaps taking it out only for special occasions, and use your new vegan bags as everyday accessories. Don't feel guilty about selling your old leather skirts and fur collars, or donating animal-based clothing to charity—yes, it means that someone will still be wearing it, but the garment will have been fully used by the time it's disposed of in a landfill. Also, the buyer of your item might have bought it instead of buying a new leather item, which discourages the production of even more animal-derived fashion items. Plus, the proceeds from that garment will go to charity, which should help to alleviate your guilt.

HOW AND WHERE TO ACQUIRE ITEMS THAT FIT YOUR NEW VEGAN STYLE

This is the fun part. As lost as you may feel in the shopping jungle once you start looking for alternatives to the clothing you've always worn, it can be exciting to discover new sources of fashion inspiration and define your new vegan style. The Internet is your best friend here: get familiar with online shops (see the brand directory on page 239) and check out vegan fashion bloggers for inspiration. Many of your favorite department stores will have vegan versions of the non-vegan items you used to wear, and you'll also discover lots of new, smaller, and quirkier ethical brands that pay attention to other values as well as animal welfare, such as workers' rights and the environment. You'll be amazed at how far your new ethical stance will take you.

THE VEGAN-OVER

TRANSITION
tips and tricks

Over time, and by talking to other people who have veganized their wardrobes, I've acquired some tricks that will make the transition easier and quicker—and that will ensure that you love your new, compassionate wardrobe more than you ever did your old one.

DONATE YOUR FUR

Grandma left you her old fur coat? Clueless but well-meaning relatives presented you with the unwanted gift of a fur item? Fur gifts often come from the idea that fur is a status item—the person who gave you the gift probably didn't mean any harm, and ethical concerns were the last thing on their mind. After the awkward moment has passed, it's time to start thinking about what to do with the dead animal now hanging in your wardrobe. Believe it or not, old or unwanted fur can be put to good use—one that doesn't involve your wearing it.

You can't bring those animals back or undo all the horrors they suffered, but PETA's fur donation program has helped animals in shelters get new bedding, kept homeless people warm on cold winter nights, and even been sent to refugee camps. So, don't throw out your old pelt—donate it to a good cause instead. That way, the animals' deaths won't have been completely in vain.

In the United States, Born Free Foundation has an annual "Fur for the Animals" fur drive—but, due to overwhelming response, they have now suspended the program. That just goes to show how people's attitudes are changing as compassion takes the place of vanity in their lives and wardrobes—and how much fur is still in existence that people want to get rid of!

LEARN ABOUT HIGH-QUALITY FAUX LEATHER

Not all vegan leathers are made equal. Back in the day, it was a given that real leather was superior to faux materials, but those days are long gone thanks to fashion innovation. Many modern vegan materials are light-years away from the "pleather" of the past. First of all, stay away from PVC—it's an environmental nightmare, and many ethically inclined brands steer clear of it. Polyurethane (PU) is slightly less harmful to the environment. It's also more breathable and adjusts to body temperature quicker—no more sweating in sticky faux leather.

The key characteristics to look for when shopping for a better fake

TEXTURE

You want a little bit of grain and a matte surface—smooth and shiny are quick giveaways for fake.

A GOOD FIT

Step away from anything too short, too tight, or too roomy. Fit is a tricky thing, but it's worth shopping around until you find The One. Check the fit around the shoulders and the length of the arms and body to find your fit.

WEIGHT

A good leather jacket is often a little bit heavier. If the fabric is too flimsy, it won't give you that sturdy biker feel.

PHASE THINGS OUT

When switching to a vegan diet, many of us phased out animal products one by one instead of going cold turkey (although I have such respect for those who went vegan overnight). It's often the same with clothing. Don't feel guilty for still having the odd pair of leather shoes in your wardrobe—most of us weren't born or raised vegan, so you can hardly be blamed for following what you were taught for the majority of your life. What you can do is some research to make sure everything you buy from now on is cruelty-free. Wear those shoes until they fall apart (they will, even if the label proudly proclaims "genuine leather") and then replace them with a brand-new and shiny vegan pair to be proud of.

You will get questions along your journey about why you're still wearing leather or wool. Explain that you're phasing out animal-based clothes and that you're on a journey, and more progress will come with time. Many lifestyle changes are gradual transitions. Don't let that push you off your path.

EXPLORE NEW BRANDS

Creating a vegan wardrobe is the perfect excuse for hours and hours of online browsing to discover the sure-to-be-cult brands that will elevate your new, compassionate wardrobe to unexpected heights of chic.

The Bespoke option

Whether you're looking for a wear-it-forever dress or a dress you'll wear only once (on your wedding day), another option is having a one-of-a-kind garment made using vegan fabric. Bespoke couture design studio Tammam in London focuses on sustainable and vegan fabric, specializing in gorgeous gowns that are the opposite of throwaway fast fashion.

LEARN ABOUT ECO MATERIALS

Once again, not all vegan materials are the same. Just because it's good for the animals, it (unfortunately) doesn't mean it's automatically better for the planet—as I previously mentioned, PVC is a vegan material, but it's hardly an eco-friendly one. The upside: there are many natural materials, some upcycled, that are much better for the planet than animal-derived clothing whose production creates toxic pollution and causes extensive damage to land and waterways.

In a time when more and more people are concerned with the origins of what they wear, innovation is taking center stage in the vegan fashion arena—to ensure that the new substitutes for leather are as environmentally friendly as they can be, which often means working creatively with natural fibers instead of petroleum-based synthetics. Here are a few up-and-comers that might outshine leather in the years to come.

MUSHROOM LEATHER

One of the newest innovations in the game is MuSkin, a biodegradable vegan "leather" extracted from mushroom caps. MuSkin is produced using chemical-free tanning, entirely without the use of toxic substances, and is worked to obtain a suede- or leatherlike finish.

CORK

This completely natural, recyclable, and renewable material (see page 60) might not be your first choice when you think of fashion, but recently, vegan brands have interpreted cork in entirely new and visually interesting ways. Examples include Jentil, a French brand that creates men's and women's accessories in a variety of colors; Portuguese brand Corkor with their collection of clutches, handbags, and wallets; and Canadian label Rok Cork, offering sustainable accessories produced ethically in Portugal.

KOMBUCHA LEATHER

If trendy, healthy, and somewhat obscure food ingredients are your thing, you may have heard of kombucha, a fermented tea originating in China that has taken the health-food scene by storm in the last few years due to its probiotic and antioxidant properties. However, this magical ingredient has another potential use: it can be used to create a leatherlike fabric. The cellulose fibers that are a by-product of the tea can be dried and made into fashion accessories. It's still in the works and not ready for purchase just yet, but watch this space.

WINE LEATHER

Winner of H&M Foundation's Global Change Award of 2017, Italian company Vegea makes a vegan material made from leftover grape skins, stalks, and seeds from wine production. The company and its leader, Rosa Rossella Longobardo, noted that each year, thirteen million tons of waste are generated from the wine industry, so they set out to recycle this waste into an exciting new material that might save countless animal lives.

PINEAPPLE LEATHER

This vegan-friendly material, created by Dr. Carmen Hijosa of Ananas Anam, is made from waste pineapple-leaf fibers that are a by-product of pineapple harvesting, meaning that no extra resources such as land, water, fertilizers, or pesticides are used in the production of these fibers.

APPLE LEATHER

Apple leather is made from the peel, seeds, and pulp of apples, and is used by several vegan accessory brands such as bag brand Alexandra K from Poland and Italian shoe label Nemanti Milano. It's very soft and supple and 100 percent biodegradable. Danish company Apple Girl is developing an apple leather that requires only one quart of water per yard of "leather"—compared to two thousand gallons needed to make one pound of animal leather.

VEGAN STYLE

FIND OUT WHERE TO SHOP ONLINE

One beautiful discovery you'll make when you start scouring the web for animal-friendly fashion is that ASOS has a filter that lets you search for non-leather items. And that NET-A-PORTER.com is actually a fur-free retailer. And that iconic designer brands like Chanel no longer sell fur and exotic skins. And, once you're ready for some serious all-vegan shopping, ethical multibrand retailers like Modavanti (page 195), Bead & Reel (page 158), and Unicorn Goods (page 170) offer plenty of beautiful cruelty-free clothing, and visiting their sites will free you from having to read labels, as everything on these sites is vegan-friendly.

For some inspiration, and to see how easy vegan dressing can be, check out the #veganfashion or #whatveganswear hashtags on Instagram to find out what cruelty-free fashionistas around the world are wearing and where they got it. My magazine has its own hashtag, #VildaOOTD (for "outfit of the day," a popular hashtag), to celebrate vegan fashion all over the globe. Get familiar with the brands around the globe that understand vegan fashion and know how to bring it to the masses—they are the future, so knowing all about them will put you at the forefront of fashion.

Of course, budget is a concern for many, but there's no need to bankrupt yourself by shopping vegan. Shopping secondhand is a great way to indulge your love of fashion while remaining on the ethical and sustainable side. EBay is also a gold mine for vegan shopping—you can find Matt & Nat, Beyond Skin, and even Stella McCartney for a fraction of the price. Secondhand sites like Vestiaire Collective and HEWI (Hardly Ever Worn It) are also full of designer goodies at amazing prices.

THE VEGAN-OVER

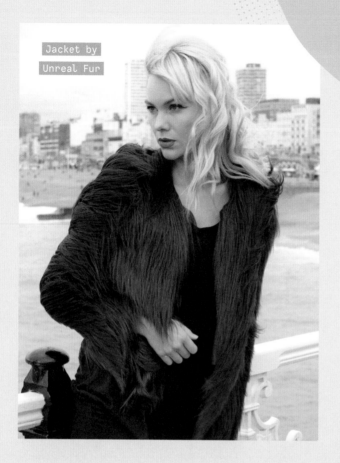

Jacket by
Unreal Fur

FUR

LEARN TO DISTINGUISH FAUX FROM THE REAL DEAL

Yup, we're talking label-reading again—but as a vegan, you're probably already used to that. Sometimes things are unlabeled and sometimes labels aren't very clear, so get used to doing some nosing around to find out if that faux fur really is just that, or if those shoes are real leather.

How to know whether your fur is faux

Why is it important to check whether your fur is faux? There have been several instances when real fur was mislabeled and sold as faux, and due to the low price point, most customers were certain that these products were indeed made from faux fur. As China has a thriving dog- and cat-fur industry with pelts sold at low prices, this could very well have meant that this fur came from a cat or a dog. So, the next time you're unsure, try these three tricks:

IT'S IN THE TIPS

Carefully look at the tip of each hair on your coat. Animal hair typically tapers at the end (like human hair), whereas faux fur remains the same width. This isn't a sure-fire indicator, though; if the hair has been sheared or plucked, it does not necessarily taper.

BURN IT

Inherited a fur coat from your mom and you're not sure whether it's real or faux? Do the burn test: pluck a few hairs from the coat and light them on fire. Real fur burns the way human hair would, whereas faux fur has a plasticky smell when burned. Captain Obvious adds: This is, of course, not one to try in a shop!

CHECK THE BASE

The surest way to see if your fur is real or faux is by looking at the base, where the hair meets the backing. Faux fur is sewn onto a fabric backing, and you'll see the threadwork, whereas real fur has a hide backing.

THE VEGAN-OVER

LEATHER

Often you'll know that the leather you're looking at in a shop or online is real because the brand will tell you—a feature like "genuine leather" is often proudly displayed on the garment in one way or another, be it a symbol (see page 22) or the wording clearly spelled out on the label or product page. But just in case you're unsure, here are some clues that the leather is, in fact, fake:

CHECK FOR TEXTURE

Real leather is often grainier than faux, which tends to be smoother all over.

DO THE PIERCE TEST

If you already own the garment, try piercing the leather with a needle. Real leather is harder to pierce than faux.

SHOES: READ THE LABEL

It's not always obvious whether shoes or other accessories are made from real leather or faux alternatives. When it comes to shoes, there's an easy way to tell. When you're in the shop, read the label. Even if it doesn't say what material the shoe is made from, it will have symbols on the sole that you can use as a guide. The key is to check whether you see a diamond symbol or one that looks like a cowhide. The diamond means that the material is faux, whereas the cowhide signals that the leather came from an animal. Sometimes there will be a net-like design that stands for "other man-made materials."

LEARN HOW TO REPLACE

Phasing things out of your wardrobe can be daunting. What fabrics and materials are good substitutes for the animal-based clothing that you're used to? Relying too heavily on synthetics can also be harmful to the environment, so always prioritize natural fabrics such as cotton, linen, or bamboo, or innovative fabrics like Tencel, Piñatex, and other natural fabrics that are kind to both animals and the environment.

LEATHER

Replace with faux leather, preferably from a natural source (although it will probably take a few years before these truly hit the market) such as mushroom leather, Piñatex, kombucha leather (see page 222), or Vegea.

SILK

Replace with cotton (preferably organic), bamboo, Tencel, linen, or recycled synthetics.

FUR

Replace with faux fur or a wool-free coat in recycled synthetics.

WOOL/ANGORA

Replace with cotton (preferably organic), cotton blends, or recycled synthetics.

DOWN

Replace with technical tissues such as PrimaLoft, Flocus, Thermal R, Omni-Heat, or Cocona.

THE VEGAN-OVER

LASTLY...
lead by example

As vegans, we're constantly sending a message to others about our lifestyle. Whether we like it or not, we are the image of veganism to the non-vegans we come across. So, make a habit of dressing well and truly put your heart into expressing your personality through style. That way, you'll help to get rid of the clichéd image of vegan fashion and make way for a new, more inspiring image of veganism. And that's what we all need.

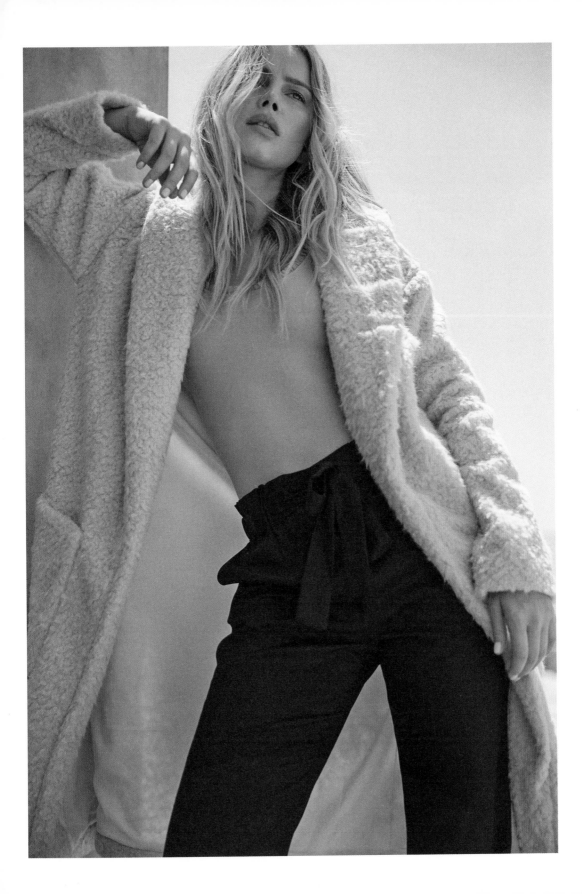

CONCLUSION

What does the world hold for vegan fashion?

As I type this, I'm wearing my faux-leather trousers and my ankle boots from By Blanch. My Jill Milan bag lies on the table next to me, with my Beyond Skin wallet falling out of it. I'm wrapped up in a cozy, wool-free cable-knit sweater (it's pretty chilly), and no part of my outfit contains animal-derived substances.

And I'm not the only one. Through the work that I do, I've met countless people who have not only removed animal flesh and derivatives from their diets but also animal skins from their wardrobes. It was as much of a no-brainer for them as it was for me, and, in this day and age, their choice is becoming more and more accepted. They have no difficulties shopping for cutting-edge clothing that's completely vegan.

My friends and I are in glamorous company: actresses like Natalie Portman are asking film sets to provide vegan shoes; brands like Gucci, Hugo Boss, and Calvin Klein are fur-free; and designers like Marni are experimenting with vegan bags. Smaller vegan brands such as Jill Milan and Beyond Skin are worn by celebrities on red carpets. Vegan fashion is hot—hotter than it's ever been.

Real fur is becoming obsolete as the quality of faux fur has risen to rival the real deal. London fashion brand Shrimps, founded by designer Hannah Weiland, is one of the hottest tickets at London Fashion Week. Designer houses like Gucci, Versace, Armani, Michael Kors, and Jimmy Choo have all gone proudly fur-free. Australian brand Unreal Fur is dressing bloggers and influencers in their creative and colorful faux furs. Faux is fierce, and real fur is officially dead.

Angora wool and mohair (goat fur) has almost completely disappeared from the department stores following animal rights campaigns to ban it. Brands like H&M, Gap, ASOS, Topshop,

Benetton, and Zara have all implemented bans on these materials, and they're both becoming virtually impossible to find in most fashion chains. All because of the compassionate actions of concerned shoppers.

Leather is deemed by many to be the final frontier—a symbol of fashion and quality. Quite the contrary, after finding out more about the damage that animal agriculture does to the environment, more and more meat-reducers (those who are consciously trying to reduce their meat consumption) are also giving up leather, and brands are looking for new ways to mimic the material without killing animals. Most fabric innovation today isn't happening in the world of leather or other animal-derived materials—it's vegan textiles that are leading the way. Hence innovation in the form of leatherlike fabrics made from pineapples, wine grapes, mushrooms, and kombucha, just to name a few. Real leather is still a very present factor in the fashion world, but these futuristic fabrics are set to take over, due to their eco-credentials and cruelty-free appeal. And the ultimate seal of approval came from Fashion Week itself—namely Helsinki Fashion Week, which implemented a ban on all animal leather starting in 2019.

"Environmentally sustainable" is more than a buzz term—it's a new way of determining quality. Gone are the days when status was set by how much you spent on your clothes. The new status symbol is knowing #whomadeyourclothes—but also what your clothes are made from and being well-informed about the journey that sweater or jacket made before it ended up in your wardrobe. Leather is very difficult, if not impossible, to trace back to its origins. This has led many consumers to ask questions about animal-derived clothing and whether that "genuine leather" label is indeed worth it. Increasingly, the answer is no.

CONCLUSION

Today's fashion industry is a revolutionary affair. It engages in political and social issues such as feminism and human rights. It speaks out loud rather than quietly whispering. It's far from the status-obsessed affair of the 1980s or the I-couldn't-care-less attitude of the '90s. The contemporary fashion scene is concerned and it's conscious. And so, it's only predictable and logical that animal skins are, and will be, slowly but surely phased out of fashion.

As interest in vegan living skyrockets, the clothing industry is bound to feel the effects of a rising consciousness that inspires more and more people to stop eating and wearing animals. Just because something has been done a certain way for hundreds of years doesn't mean it's justified or supposed to stay the same, and the aforementioned new leather alternatives are just a small fraction of all the innovation that's coming—the sky's the limit.

And the bit that brands are increasingly getting right? The style factor. Many non-vegans are buying vegan fashion just because it looks good—possibly even better than the mainstream fashion they're used to. You don't have to be a vegan to wear Shrimps's eye-catching faux furs, and I've met many non-vegans sporting the beautiful creations of Hannah Weiland just because they're sublimely gorgeous and on-trend.

I started *Vilda* magazine because there were very few online voices that spoke to a vegan consumer from a fashion-forward point of view, and I wanted to be one of them. I wanted to create a beautiful, luxuriously glossy space that was curated and cool, and offered inspiration to vegans and those curious about a vegan-friendly way of living. I wanted *Vilda* to be read by vegans and non-vegans alike, and I wanted it to be a source of inspiration first and foremost.

To attract the client who is not driven by ethical motivations but by a pure love of fashion, brands need to speak their language— collections need to have the "have to have it" appeal beyond the ethics and moral values. Fashion is a visual means of expression, and designers are realizing that if they're going to hit the big time, their styles need more than just a vegan-friendly tag. They need the approval of the style set. A consumer base that's mainly ethically minded will sooner or later find its way to a vegan brand. But since humans are, by nature, vain creatures, the fashion factor will always lead the way when it comes to consumer choices, which is why a fashion label that doesn't wholly focus on style will never reach beyond a very niche group of customers. It's when vegan and ethical labels start to prioritize style, to hire designers from conventional fashion backgrounds, and to pay attention to trends that things shift and ethical becomes mainstream.

The challenges of vegan fashion, beyond leather, include bringing eco-conscious substitutes for wool into the mainstream. When days get chillier, we need to turn to organic cotton blends, hemp, soybean fiber, Tencel, and other sustainable and kind options. Wool is still viewed as an eco-friendly material, and the idea that "sheep need to be sheared" dies hard, but animal-rights campaigns documenting multiple cases of abuse in sheep sheds across the planet are challenging that perception. In 2015, Patagonia famously cut ties with their wool supplier, the Ovis 21 networks in Argentina, following a PETA investigation that found horrific conditions and violent treatment of the sheep in the network's facilities. Stella McCartney also dropped Ovis 21 and is now looking into switching to vegan wool. My money is on her being the game-changer on the runways, and when that change arrives, vegans will smile, knowing that another pioneering designer led the way.

When asked about the future of vegan fashion at PETA's vegan fashion show in January 2017, VAUTE founder Leanne Mai-ly Hilgart says, "I just don't believe that living creatures belong in business. . . . We've made everything in factories and industrialized everything into machine parts—and animals are not machine parts. It's inevitable that there will be a point where everything will be vegan."

For the sake of the billion animals who are killed in the leather industry every year, for the sake of Bangladesh's tannery workers, for the sake of the fifty million animals killed each year for their fur, for the sake of our planet, I hope that Leanne is right.

THANK YOU

To my team at Murdoch Books—Corinne Roberts, Lou Johnson, Julie Mazur Tribe, Andrea O'Connor, Megan Pigott, Madeleine Kane, Justine Harding, Carol Warwick, and Lou Playfair—it has been a pleasure to share this adventure with you. Thank you so much for taking a chance on an unknown first-time author—and with a niche topic, at that. I've learned so much from working with you.

To all the photographers whose images appear in this book: thank you infinitely for lending your wonderful work to this project. Without your photos, I doubt very much that anyone would have looked twice at this book!

All the designers, influencers, and other tastemakers I've had the immense pleasure of interviewing for this project: I'm in awe of your work. Thank you for being advocates for cruelty-free fashion, beauty, and lifestyle.

The team at PETA and its international affiliates: thank you for being my transition into working in animal rights full-time. I will forever be proud of working for such a revolutionary, groundbreaking organization. Let's keep changing the world together.

My first-ever mentor in journalism, Camilla Bjorkman: thank you for sharing your skills, wisdom, and insight to help make me the writer I always hoped—but never dared believe—that I could be.

A special thanks to *Marie Claire* magazine UK, Miranda McMinn, and Poppy Dinsey for playing a crucial role in bringing *Vilda* magazine to life. I owe you so much.

My husband, David Camilli, for being my biggest supporter and my rock to lean on. There were so many times when I had you and no one else, and there is no way I would have been holding this book in my hands if I didn't have you with me on this ride. I love you beyond words.

My family: my mom, Zoia; my dad, Andrei; my sisters Sofie and Liza—thanks for your constant encouragement and faith in my abilities (and for putting up with my whining!). You're my everything.

My dear friends Johanna Picano, Angela Susini, Karen Denton, Giulia Panna, Jacky Moya, Laura De Filippo, and everyone else who was by my side as I worked on this project: I love you.

A special thanks to my only writer friend, Stefano De Martino. You have been my light in the darkness on so many occasions. I don't know if this book could ever have happened without your tireless support.

The team behind *Vilda* magazine: I'm so, so thankful to have you by my side and so grateful for your skills, talent, and time. Thank you for helping me see my dream come to life on a screen.

Lastly, this book is dedicated to the readers of *Vilda* magazine. Thank you so much to everyone who has ever visited my website and to those who have contributed to our amazing journey. This book is for you, and I hope you stay with us as we continue to be a voice for a compassionate future, in fashion and beyond.

INDEX

VEGAN STYLE

DIRECTORY OF BRANDS AND RETAILERS

TILLER PRESS

An Imprint of Simon & Schuster, Inc.
1230 Avenue of the Americas
New York, NY 10020

First Tiller Press hardcover edition November 2019

TILLER PRESS and colophon are trademarks of
Simon & Schuster, Inc.

For information about special discounts for
bulk purchases, please contact Simon &
Schuster Special Sales at 1-866-506-1949 or
business@simonandschuster.com.

The Simon & Schuster Speakers Bureau can bring
authors to your live event. For more information
or to book an event, contact the Simon & Schuster
Speakers Bureau at 1-866-248-3049 or visit our
website at www.simonspeakers.com.

Manufactured in China

10 9 8 7 6 5 4 3 2 1

Library of Congress Cataloging-in-Publication
Data has been applied for.

ISBN 978-1-9821-3981-0
ISBN 978-1-9821-3982-7 (ebook)

Publisher: Corinne Roberts
Editorial Manager: Julie Mazur Tribe
Design Manager: Megan Pigott
Designer: Madeleine Kane
Editor: Andrea O'Connor
Production Director: Lou Playfair

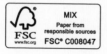

Photographer credits: 9, 157: Lorena Sturlese;
11: Sharron Goodyear; 19, 45: Per Norberg (styling by
Anna Fernmo, modelled by Annika Marie); 32: Valery
Rizzo; 34, 224: David Camilli; 40 (right), 168,
169: EG Photography (Emma Groenenboom),
© University of Applied Photography; 47: Robin
Griffin; 49, 215: Federica Dall'Orso; 58: Landa
Penders; 66: Moanalani Jeffrey Photography; 67
(left): Lance Staedler (modelled by Kristina Szabo);
71: Helani Sarath Kumara; 77: © WR8; 78: © Chris
Swoszowski; 90–91: M.A.S. Photography; 104: © Line
Klein; 109, 118, 123, 196, 229, back cover (second
from top): Trever Hoehne; 127: Nik Merkulo
(Shutterstock); 135: all rights reserved © Nic
Davidson (bushy.com.au); 136: Picasa; 146: Emma
Weatherby; 150: Christina Pippin; 160: Peter Adams;
162: Helani Sarath Kumara; 164: Amanda Valentine;
172, 193: © Brandon Michael Kelly; 174: Kalie
Johnstone; 175: Amar Bhakta/Seven Islands
Photography (makeup by Joseph Adivari, hair by
Suzy Balderas, styling by Komie Vora and Meg
Vora); 184: Eric Mirbach; 189: Jordan Curtis Hughes.

Image credits: The publisher also wishes to thank
the following individuals and organizations who
generously supplied photography.
Pages 6–7, 62, 171, back cover (bottom): Angela Roi;
8: Shelly Vella; 25: Monkee Genes; 29, 30, 145, 195:
Reformation; 33: Woocoa; 37: Beyond Skin; 40
(left), 65: Matt & Nat; 51, 74: By Blanch; 52, 81, 181:
Bourgeois Boheme; 67 (product shots): Jill Milan;
72: Vanita Bagri; 73: LaBante; 79: Bebe Mehr; 80:
Alicia Lai; 92–93: Suszi Saunders; 100: Chloe Bullock;
102, back cover (second from bottom): The Nomad
Society; 112: Eden DiBianco; 124: Madeline Alcott;
131, 147, back cover (top): Marsha Derevianko; 140:
Elvis & Kresse; 158: Sica Schmitz; 166: Julia Koch;
170: Cayla Mackey; 206: Ovide

Color reproduction by Splitting Image Colour
Studio Pty Ltd, Clayton, Victoria
Printed by C & C Offset Printing Co. Ltd., China